WB 18

Self-assessment for the MRCP Part 2 Written Paper:
Volume 3 Data Interpretation

Self-assessment for the MRCP Part 2 Written Paper:
Volume 3
Data Interpretation

Balwinder Bajaj BSc MRCP PhD
Consultant Physician and Cardiologist
Royal Oldham Hospital
Oldham

Narinder Bajaj MA MRCP PhD
Honorary Lecturer in Neurology
Specialist Registrar in Neurology
National Hospital for Neurology
London

Karim Meeran MD FRCP
Consultant Endocrinologist
Charing Cross and Hammersmith Hospitals
London

EDITORIAL ADVISOR

Huw Beynon BSc MD FRCP
Consultant Physician and Rheumatologist
The Royal Free Hospital School of Medicine
Royal Free Hospital
London

Blackwell
Science

© 2002 by Blackwell Science Ltd
a Blackwell Publishing Company
Editorial Offices:
Osney Mead, Oxford OX2 0EL, UK
 Tel: +44 (0)1865 206206
108 Cowley Road, Oxford OX4 1JF, UK
 Tel: +44 (0)1865 791100
Blackwell Publishing USA, 350 Main Street, Malden, MA 02148-5018, USA
 Tel: +1 781 388 8250
Iowa State Press, a Blackwell Publishing Company, 2121 State Avenue, Ames, Iowa 50014-8300, USA
 Tel: +1 515 292 0140
Blackwell Munksgaard, Nørre Søgade 35, PO Box 2148, Copenhagen, DK-1016, Denmark
 Tel: +45 77 33 33 33
Blackwell Publishing Asia, 54 University Street, Carlton, Victoria 3053, Australia
 Tel: +61 (0)3 9347 0300
Blackwell Verlag, Kurfürstendamm 57, 10707 Berlin, Germany
 Tel: +49 (0)30 32 79 060
Blackwell Publishing, 10 rue Casimir Delavigne, 75006 Paris, France
 Tel: +33 1 53 10 33 10

The Blackwell Publishing logo is a trade mark of Blackwell Publishing Ltd

First published 2002
Reprinted 2003

Catalogue records for this title are available from the Library of Congress and the British Library

ISBN 0-632-06442-0

Set in 8/10 Frutiger Condensed by Best-set Typesetter Ltd., Hong Kong
Printed and bound in Great Britain by MPG Books Ltd, Bodmin Cornwall

For further information on Blackwell Publishing, visit our website:
www.blackwellpublishing.com

Contents

vii   **Preface**

ix   **Normal values**

1   **Questions**

201   **EMQs**

217   **Listing by specialty**

219   **Index**

Preface

This book is part of a series of three, designed to provide a revision course for the written part of the MRCP examination. Together with Volume 1 (Picture Tests) and Volume 2 (Case Histories), they comprise a significant volume of work giving ample coverage of the MRCP syllabus.

The 100 data questions contained in this volume encompass the full range of general medical problems encountered in hospital practice. Cardiology data is well represented with electrocardiography, echocardiography and cardiac catheterisation questions. These latter subjects are often neglected in current MRCP orientated texts. The final chapter in this volume is devoted to EMQ type questions: these are increasingly in use for the MRCP examination.

The writing of this text has been a lengthy one and we would like to thank all members of our respective families for their support and patience during this time. NPSB and BPSB would especially like to thank their father (a long established author) for his words of wisdom.

NPSB, BPSB, KM 2001.

Normal values

Chemical pathology

Sodium (Na)	135–145 mmol/l
Potassium (K)	3.5–5.0 mmol/l
Urea (U)	3.3–6.7 mmol/l
Creatinine (Cr)	45–120 µmol/l
Bicarbonate (HCO_3^-)	22–30 mmol/l
Calcium (Ca)	2.2–2.67 mmol/l
Phosphate (PO_4)	0.8–1.5 mmol/l
Magnesium (Mg)	0.7–1.1 mmol/l
Copper (Cu)	11–22 µmol/l
Caeruloplasmin	0.20–0.60 g/l
Chloride (Cl)	95–105 mmol/l
Cholesterol (Ch)	3.6–7.8 mmol/l
Triglyceride (TG)	0.8–2.1 mmol/l
Creatinine phosphokinase (CPK)	
Male	17–148 IU/l
Female	10–79 IU/l
Urate	180–420 µmol/l
Glucose (fasting)	4.5–5.8 mmol/l
Glycosylated haemoglobin (HbA_{1C})	3.8–6.4%
Lactate	0.6–1.8 mmol/l
Total protein (TP)	60–80 g/l
Albumin (Alb)	35–50 g/l
Bilirubin (Bili)	3–20 µmol/l
Alkaline phosphatase (Alk P)	30–130 IU/l
Alanine amino transferase (ALT)	5–30 IU/l
Aspartate transaminase (AST)	10–50 IU/l
Gamma glutamyl transferase (GGT)	5–40 IU/l
Amylase	46–330 IU/l
Globulin (Glob)	25–35 g/l
Alphafetoprotein	<10 IU/ml
Angiotensin-converting enzyme	204–358 U/l
Plasma osmolality	275–295 mosmol/l

Endocrine tests

Total serum thyroxine (T4)	58–174 nmol/l
Total serum triiodothyronine (T3)	1.2–3.1 nmol/l
Free serum thyroxine (FT4)	13–30 pmol/l
Free triiodothyronine (FT3)	2.8–7.1 pmol/l
Thyroid stimulating hormone (TSH)	0.3–6.0 mU/l
Testosterone	
Male	9–35 nmol/l
Female	0.9–3.1 nmol/l

Cortisol
    (0900 hours)   280–700 nmol/l
    (2400 hours)   80–280 nmol/l

Prolactin
    Male   <450 mU/l
    Female   <600 mU/l
Adrenocorticotrophic hormone (ACTH)   <10–80 ng/l
Growth hormone (GH)   <20 mU/l (<5 ng/ml after 75 g oral glucose challenge)

Urinary values

Urine copper	15–78 μmol/24 h (0.01–0.06 mg/24 h)
Urine vanillyl mandelic acid (VMA)	5–35 μmol/24 h
Urine creatinine	0.13–0.22 mmol/kg body weight, daily
Urine protein (quantitative)	<0.15 g/24 h
Urine sodium	50–125 mmol/l
	100–250 mmol/24 h

Blood gas measurements (room air)

pO_2	11.2–14 kPa
pCO_2	4.6–6.0 kPa
pH	7.35–7.45
Base excess	0 ± 2 mmol/l

Haematology

Haemoglobin (Hb)	
Male	13–18 g/dl
Female	11.5–15 g/dl
White cell count (WCC)	$4.0–11.0 \times 10^9$/l
Red cell count (RBC)	$3.8–5.8 \times 10^{12}$/l
Packed cell volume (PCV) (haematocrit)	
Male	0.4–0.54
Female	0.37–0.47
Mean corpuscular volume (MCV)	79.0–96.0 fl
Mean corpuscular haemoglobin (MCH)	27.0–32.0 pg
Mean corpuscular haemoglobin concentration (MCHC)	31.5–36.0 g/dl
Platelet (Plt)	$150–450 \times 10^9$/l
Reticulocyte count	0.2–2%
Prothrombin time (PT)	12–16 s
International normalized ratio (INR)	0.90–1.20
Activated partial thromboplastin time (APTT)	23–33 s
Thrombin time (TT)	15–19 s
Fibrinogen	1.5–4.5 g/l

Vitamin B_{12}	180–1100 ng/l (150–675 pmol/l)
Folate (serum)	4.0–18.0 µg/l (5–63 nmol/l)
Folate (red cell)	160–640 µg/l
Iron (Fe)	13–32 µmol/l (50–150 µg/dl)
Iron binding capacity (TIBC)	40–80 µmol/l (250–410 µg/dl)
Ferritin	15–250 µg/l (5.8–120 nmol/l)
Transferrin	1.2–2 g/l
Neutrophils	$2.50–7.50 \times 10^9$/l
Lymphocytes	$1.30–4.00 \times 10^9$/l
Monocytes	$0.0–1.00 \times 10^9$/l
Eosinophils	$0.04–0.40 \times 10^9$/l
Basophils	$0.0–0.10 \times 10^9$/l
Erythrocyte sedimentation rate	
Male	age/2 mm/h
Female	age + 10/2 mm/h

Immunology

Immunoglobulin G (IGG)	7.0–18.6 g/l
Immunoglobulin M (IGM)	0.49–2.0 g/l
Immunoglobulin A (IGA)	0.78–4.8 g/l
Anti-double stranded DNA titre (dsDNA)	<60 IU/ml
Anti-mitochondrial antibody	10–47 µmol/l
Complement (C3)	0.55–1.30 g/l
Complement (C4)	0.20–0.60 g/l
C-reactive protein	<10 mg/l

Cerebrospinal fluid

Protein	0.15–0.4 g/l
Glucose	2.8–4.5 g/l
Cells	<5 white/red cells mm^{-3}
Pressure	70–180 mm H_2O

Haemodynamic normal values
(pressure measurements in mmHg)

Systemic arterial

Peak systolic/end-diastolic	100–140/60–90
Mean	70–105

Left ventricular

Peak systolic/end diastolic	100–140/3–12

Left atrial (or pulmonary capillary wedge)

Mean	2–12
a wave	3–10
v wave	3–15

Pulmonary artery

Peak systolic/end diastolic	15–30/4–14
Mean	9–17

Right ventricular

Peak systolic/end diastolic	15–30/2–7

Right atrial

Mean	2–6
a wave	2–8
v wave	2–7

Resistances [(dyn.s)/cm^5]

Systemic vascular resistance	700–1600
Total pulmonary resistance	100–300
Pulmonary vascular resistance	30–130

Flows

Cardiac index (l/min m^{-2})	2.4–3.8
Stroke index (mm/beat m^{-2})	30–65

A 56-year-old female smoker presented with orthopnoea, exertional chest pain and dyspnoea. On examination, she was in controlled atrial fibrillation, had an ejection systolic murmur and a mid-diastolic murmur with an opening snap. There was peripheral pitting oedema and bilateral basal crackles at both pulmonary bases.

A transthoracic echocardiogram was performed and reported as follows:

Left ventricular ejection fraction 28%.

Aortic and mitral valves heavily calcified.

Left atrial size 5.6 cm.

Aortic stenosis, peak pressure gradient 26 mmHg.

Mitral valve area 0.7 cm^2.

A What is the aetiology of this woman's biventricular cardiac failure?

B What medications would you recommend?

A Mild aortic stenosis and critical mitral stenosis. As the normal mitral valve area is 4–6 cm^2, a mitral valve area of less than 1 cm^2 is indicative of critical valve stenosis. Underlying ischaemic heart disease would also need to be excluded, although chest pain *per se* may occur as a feature of mitral stenosis and may indeed be indistinguishable from that produced by coronary artery disease.

B Diuretics and anticoagulants.

A 26-year-old nulliparous female presents with a history of recurrent pulmonary emboli. She is not taking any regular medication and is a non-smoker. There is no family history of thrombo-embolic disease. There were no significant findings on physical examination.

Her haematological investigations are shown below [PT, TT, APTT and KCCT are expressed as a ratio of the control value (shown as the denominator)]:

Prothrombin time (PT) 15 s/14 s, Thrombin time (TT) 15 s/14 s, Activated partial thromboplastin time (APTT) 36 s/30 s, Kaolin-cephalin clotting time (KCCT) 65 s/38 s, Anti-thrombin III levels: 94% of normal

Protein S and C levels normal

Parts Normal Plasma	10	8	5	2	0
Parts Sample Plasma	0	2	5	8	10
APTT (s):	39	45	57	64	68

A What phenomenon is demonstrated by these results?

B What additional tests would you require in reaching a diagnosis?

A Lupus anticoagulant.
This patient's coagulation studies demonstrate a prolongation of her APTT and KCCT. The dilution of the patient's plasma with normal plasma does not correct the coagulation defect, which thereby excludes the deficiency of a clotting factor and favours the presence of an inhibitor of coagulation, e.g. antiphospholipid antibodies. This was first described in the plasma of patients with SLE and therefore termed the lupus anticoagulant. This is a misnomer because a hypercoagulable state ensues resulting in thrombo-embolic events (both arterial and venous). It is now believed that the basis for the lupus anticoagulant is antiphospholipid antibodies.

B Platelet count, dsDNA and antiphospholipid antibody titres.
In patients with clinical SLE, there is a statistical association between the presence of the lupus anticoagulant/antiphospholipid antibodies and the occurrence of thromboses, neurological disorders (e.g. cerebrovascular events), thrombocytopenia and recurrent foetal loss. In the absence of SLE, i.e. no photosensitive rash, polyserositis, renal disease, high titre for dsDNA antibodies, etc., these patients may have the primary phospholipid syndrome. A spectrum of disease exists between these two forms. Congenital deficiencies of antithrombin III, protein S and C are comparatively rare. The commonest of this group of disorders is activated protein C resistance (factor V Leiden). Activated protein C inhibits coagulation by proteolytic cleavage of factor Va and VIIIa (both procoagulant proteins). Protein C resistance may result from a mutation in the activated protein C cleavage site of factor V (factor V Leiden), resulting in thrombophilia.

A 37-year-old male was admitted following a witnessed seizure. He had no previous history of epilepsy, had been diagnosed as being HIV positive four years earlier, and his CD4 count two months previously was 7 cell/µl (normal range 350–880 cells/µl). He was on treatment for *Mycobacterium avium intracellulare*, together with warfarin for a previous pulmonary embolus.

On examination he was drowsy, and had oral candidiasis and anal warts. Clinical examination was otherwise unremarkable and there was no neurological focus.

The following results are available:

Sodium 140 mmol/l, potassium 4.1 mmol/l, urea 4.1 mmol/l, creatinine 81 µmol/l, glucose 4.0 mmol/l

Hb 14.1 g/dl, Plts 109×10^9/l, WCC 2.9×10^9/l, neutrophils 1.3×10^9/l, lymphocytes 0.8×10^9/l

INR 2.6.

CT brain: oedematous brain with midline shift to the right.

CSF: 13 white cells (25% polymorphs, 75% lymphocytes), 25 red blood cells, glucose 2.6 mmol/l, protein 0.79 g/l, no organisms seen; Nigracin stain/Ziehl–Nielsen negative.

A Give a differential diagnosis for this man's presentation.

B What treatment would you start this man on?

A CMV encephalitis/ Varicella zoster encephalitis/ HIV encephalitis.

B Intravenous acyclovir or gancyclovir.
Oral dexamethasone.
Phenytoin.

The most likely diagnosis, based on the rapid onset with mild meningism, is CMV encephalitis. This is supported further by the low CD4 count and the CSF findings, which in the absence of fungae or AAFB on specific staining, would be in keeping with a viral aetiology. *Varicella zoster* encephalitis is a possibility, and in patients who are HIV positive disease may occur without the characteristic rash. HIV encephalitis has a more insidious onset and is usually present with advanced dementia. HSV encephalitis is also a possibility, but is relatively rare in the context of HIV infection. The probable diagnosis of CMV encephalitis in this case may be confirmed by culture of the CSF, urine or respiratory secretions for CMV, and PCR analysis of the CSF. An EEG would be expected to show diffuse slowing and dysrhythmia.

A 70-year-old female was referred to a medical outpatient clinic with shortness of breath on exertion for six months, which had recently begun to limit her activity. She was a smoker who had a past medical history of mitral valve replacement 10 years previously. Clinical examination was unremarkable.

A full blood count taken at her initial visit showed the following results:

Hb 8.5 g/dl, WCC 4.7×10^9/l, Plts 241×10^9/l, MCV 74 fl, MCH 23.5 pg, vitamin B_{12} 750 ng/l, serum folate 18 µg/l, red cell folate 605 µg/l, ferritin 20.6 ng/ml, ESR 10 mm/h.

Reticulocyte count: 28%.

Blood film: polychromasia.

Liver function tests: bilirubin 19 µmol/l, alkaline phosphatase 111 IU/l, ALT 21 IU/l, AST 42 IU/l, total protein 77 g/l, albumin 39 g/l, globulins 38 g/l.

A What is the most likely cause of her anaemia?

B What further tests would you request?

C How would you manage this patient?

A Mechanical valve haemolysis.
Intravascular haemolysis may occur in the presence of a mechanical heart valve (especially in the presence of a paravalvular leak).

B Fragmented red cells may be seen on the blood film.
Urinary urobilinogen (increased), urinary bilirubin (absent), serum haptoglobins (decreased or absent).

C Haematinics: ferrous sulphate, folic acid.
Blood transfusion: maintaining a normal haemoglobin is useful in maintaining a normal cardiac output, and hence reducing red cell trauma.
A replacement of the valve prosthesis may be indicated.

A 27-year-old male was admitted from an outpatient clinic for investigation of jaundice. He had a history of abdominal pain and weight loss with palpable hepatosplenomegaly. There was no history of foreign travel or intravenous drug abuse and he was not taking any regular medication. There was no relevant family history.

The initial investigations were as follows:

Hb 7.5 g/dl, WCC 8.4×10⁹/l, Plts 170×10⁹/l, MCV 109 fl, MCH 33 pg, MCHC 35 g/dl, ferritin 1200 ng/ml, vitamin B$_{12}$ 600 ng/l, serum folate 18 µg/l, red cell folate 650 µg/l.

Blood film: Polychromasia, target cells.

Bilirubin 115 µmol/l, alkaline phosphatase 150 IU/l, AST 103 IU/l, ALT 57 IU/l, total protein 70 g/l, albumin 28 g/l, globulins 45 g/l.

A What further investigations would you request?

B This man's reticulocyte count is found to be 12%. What further blood tests would you request to make a diagnosis?

A Ultrasound abdomen, hepatitis serology, clotting screen, α_1-antitrypsin levels, GGT levels and liver biopsy.

B Blood lipid and haptoglobin levels.

In a man of this age an accurate alcohol consumption history would be invaluable. He has a demonstrable macrocytosis (usually round macrocytes as opposed to the oval variety seen in the presence of megaloblastic bone marrow) and target cells (indicating liver disease). The liver function tests support this demonstrating the presence of a hyperbilirubinaemia, elevated liver transaminases and hypoalbuminaemia. Alcohol excess may cause a fatty liver, alcoholic hepatitis or liver cirrhosis. The tests mentioned above are to make the diagnosis and to exclude other possible causes of this presentation. The syndrome of alcoholic liver cirrhosis in association with hyperlipidaemia and haemolytic anaemia is known as Zieve's syndrome.

A 19-year-old male presented with a three-month history of weight loss, lethargy and polyuria. There is no relevant past medical history.

His initial investigations showed the following results:

Sodium 135 mmol/l, potassium 5.1 mmol/l, bicarbonate 4 mmol/l, urea 4 mmol/l, creatinine 110 μmol/l, random blood glucose 30 mmol/l.

Arterial blood gases: pH 7.1, pCO_2 1.6 kPa, pO_2 15.9 kPa, base excess −23 mmol/l.

Hb 16 g/dl, WCC 15×10^9/l, Plts 180×10^9/l.

A What is the diagnosis?

B What initial investigations would you request?

C What is your initial management?

D What are the possible complications of this condition and its treatment?

A Diabetic ketoacidosis.

B Urinalysis: to confirm ketonuria (rarely negative if there is a predominance of 3-hydroxybutyrate, which is not detectable by conventional dip-stick testing).
MSU.
Blood cultures.
Chest X-ray.

C Intravenous rehydration: If sodium <155 mmol/l, use 0.9% saline until the plasma glucose falls to less than 14 mmol/l, when 10% dextrose may be used with suitable potassium supplements. The urine output should be monitored. If hypotension or prerenal/renal failure is present, central venous pressure monitoring will be required.
Intravenous sliding scale of soluble insulin and monitoring of the BM stix.
Sodium bicarbonate is not used to correct the acidosis unless the pH is less than 7, when isotonic (1.26%) bicarbonate may be used to bring the pH up to (but no higher than) 7.00. The use of 8.4% bicarbonate should be banned.
Broad spectrum antibiotics: in case of infection.

D Adult respiratory distress syndrome, cerebral oedema, hypotension with acute renal failure, thrombo-embolism and gastric stasis.

An elderly male with mild hypertension was reviewed in an outpatient clinic. He presented with a history of increasing lethargy and palpitations. He had been found to be in atrial fibrillation by his general practitioner one month previously and had been digitalized. His only other medication was bendrofluazide for his hypertension. An ECG was organized and is shown below:

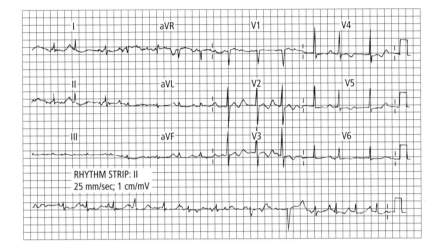

A What are the abnormalities demonstrated?

B What is the underlying cause for these changes?

C How would you manage this patient?

A Ventricular ectopic beat, ST segment depression, prominent U waves (and prolonged repolarization).

B Hypokalaemia.
The ST segment/T wave/U wave changes are typical of those seen with hypokalaemia. The cause for this, is likely to be thiazide diuretic use.

C Serum potassium assessment and subsequent supplementation will be necessary. Discontinue the digoxin as this man is already in sinus rhythm and the use of digoxin in the presence of hypokalaemia may precipitate digitoxicity.

A 60-year-old male was referred to an outpatient clinic with a three-week history of backache and declining general health. The physical examination was unremarkable, demonstrating no abdominal organomegaly and a normal rectal examination. He was a heavy smoker.

His initial investigations were as follows:

Hb 4.8 g/dl, WCC 53.8×10^9/l, Plts 140×10^9/l, MCV 78 fl, MCH 26.3 pg.

Blood film: predominantly consists of polymorphonuclear leucocytes and metamyelocytes with some nucleated red cells.

Sodium 131 mmol/l, potassium 5.6 mmol/l, bicarbonate 22 mmol/l, urea 32 mmol/l, creatinine 250 μmol/l, serum calcium 2.29 mmol/l, albumin 17 g/dl.

A What conclusions can you draw from these results?

B What is the differential diagnosis?

C What investigations would assist you further?

A Leucoerythroblastic anaemia, hypercalcaemia and renal impairment. The corrected calcium is 2.75 mmol/l because of the low albumin.

B Metastatic carcinoma with bone marrow infiltration is the most likely explanation, although multiple myeloma needs to be excluded.

C Chest X-ray, bone marrow aspirate and biopsy, urine for Bence-Jones proteins and plasma protein electrophoresis.

A leucoerythroblastic anaemia is a normochromic, normocytic anaemia characterized by the presence, in the blood, of immature myeloid cells and nucleated red cells. It may occur, as in this case, consequent to bone marrow infiltration by a metastatic tumour. Other causes include myeloma, myelofibrosis, tuberculosis, lymphoma or a lipid storage disease. Alternatively, it may occur as the bone marrow reacts to the increased demands placed upon it, e.g. during haemorrhage.

A 20-year-old office worker presented with a year-long history of a sensation that his heart was 'missing a beat'. He had a past medical history of asthma. A representative example of his 24-h tape is shown below:

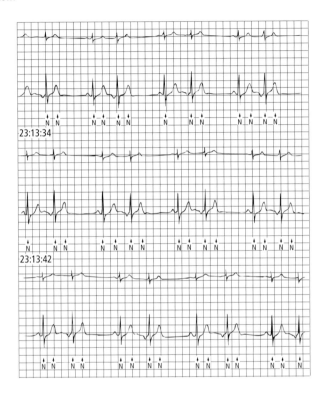

A What is the electrocardiographic abnormality illustrated?

B What additional information would you consider to be relevant in determining the cause of this abnormality?

A Atrial bigemini.
Note sinus beat followed by P wave with different axis, and then a compensatory pause.

B Atrial ectopic beats may occur in normal and diseased hearts. They are more prevalent in the presence of certain drugs, in particular sympathomimetic agents. Theophylline derivatives, as pharmacological agents or in caffeine containing beverages, may also promote their occurrence.

An 80-year-old female was admitted with a general deterioration in health. She was hypothermic, obese and had erythema *ab igne* on her legs. Her pulse was 50 min^{-1}, blood pressure 100/60 mmHg, with distant heart sounds on praecordial auscultation. Abdominal and rectal examination suggested her to be heavily constipated. She was taking thyroxine 100 µg o.d.

The results of her investigations are shown below:
Free thyroxine 14 pmol/l, TSH 76.6 mU/l.
Hb 12 g/dl, MCV 100 fl.

Choose the most likely diagnosis from those below:
(a) TSH-oma
(b) Thyroid hormone resistance
(c) Primary hypothyroidism
(d) Cold thyroid nodule
(e) Hot thyroid nodule

Comment on these results.

The clinical presentation, thyroid function tests and macrocytosis suggest primary hypothyroidism (c). This may be due to variable compliance or under-treatment. The difficulty in cardiac auscultation may relate to her obesity or may indicate the presence of a pericardial effusion. A chest X-ray is indicated.

A 25-year-old male was admitted with a history of malaise and anorexia. On examination, he was febrile, tachycardic and had several splinter haemorrhages on his fingernails. Injection marks were noted in his left antecubital fossa and left groin. Cardiac auscultation was normal.

His initial investigations are as follows:

Hb 11.2 g/dl, WCC 12×10^9/l, Plts 150×10^9/l.

Blood film: reactive lymphocytes.

Hepatitis B serology: anti-hepatitis B surface, core and 'e' antigen antibodies positive.

Hepatitis B surface antigen and 'e' antigen negative.

Hepatitis A antibody negative.

Urinalysis: microscopic haematuria.

A What further tests would you organize?

B What is this man's hepatitis B status?

C Is he infectious?

A Blood cultures, transthoracic echocardiogram and hepatitis C RNA PCR test.

B This man shows evidence of previous hepatitis B exposure but is not a carrier.

C He is not infectious.

This patient is an intravenous drug abuser. He already has evidence of exposure to the hepatitis B virus. He also needs to have hepatitis C infection excluded. In addition, intravenous drug abuse may predispose to endocarditis. The leucocytosis, pyrexia and microscopic haematuria suggest this possibility. Tricuspid valve endocarditis is the commonest valve involved in this patient group. The patient may present with obvious features of tricuspid valve involvement, although in the early stages this may not be apparent. They may present with features of pulmonary septic emboli. Acute endocarditis involving the left side of the heart may also occur.

The commonest organisms involved are *Staphylococcus aureus*, group D streptococci, *Pseudomonas aeruginosa* and *Candida*. The treatment is with suitable antibiotic or antifungal agents, although excision of the tricuspid valve (without valve replacement) may be necessary.

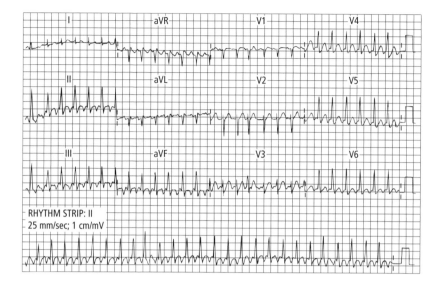

RHYTHM STRIP: II
25 mm/sec; 1 cm/mV

This patient presented with a day's history of palpitations and chest tightness. There is no past history of cardiac disease although he gives a history of significant alcohol use. The physical examination is normal. A chest radiograph shows no congestive changes. Echocardiography reveals normal left ventricular function with a structurally normal heart.

A What is the cardiac rhythm?

B How would you confirm the diagnosis?

C What would be your further management?

A Atrial flutter with 2:1 block.
This is a regular, narrow complex tachycardia with a ventricular rate of 150/min. The flutter waves are well demonstrated in V1, both before the QRS complex and superimposed upon the T waves.

B Initially attempt to confirm the diagnosis by using vagotonic manoeuvres (carotid sinus massage, breath holding or cold face towel) or adenosine, the increased atrioventricular block allowing flutter waves to be seen.
    The heart rate can be controlled using atrioventricular node blocking drugs, e.g. digoxin, verapamil, or beta-blockers. The thrombo-embolic risk can be reduced with the use of intravenous heparin. The restoration of sinus rhythm is the ultimate goal and this can be attempted using chemical or electrical means. Drugs that are capable of this include: amiodarone, flecainide and sotalol. Flecainide and sotalol are relatively contra-indicated in the presence of left ventricular dysfunction. If chemical means fail, direct current synchronized cardioversion may be necessary.

A 60-year-old female presented with nausea, vomiting, weight loss and weakness. She had a past history of long-standing breast lump with normal mammography. On examination there were no abnormal findings of note.

Her initial investigations were reported as follows:

Hb 14 g/dl, WCC 4×10^9/l, Plts 200×10^9/l, ESR 1 mm/h.

Sodium 135 mmol/l, potassium 3.9 mmol/l, bicarbonate 23 mmol/l, urea 6.9 mmol/l, creatinine 91 μmol/l.

Plasma protein electrophoresis: IgG (κ) paraproteinaemia. Normal γ-globulin levels but an abnormal protein band in the far γ region.

Serum proteins: Total proteins 70 g/l, albumin 39 g/l, globulins 31 g/l, IgG 15 g/l, IgA 1 g/l, IgM 1 g/l.

Chest X-ray: normal.

A What is the diagnosis?

B What other tests would you request?

C How would you manage this woman?

A Monoclonal gammopathy of uncertain significance (MGUS). There is no connection with her presenting symptoms.

B Urine for Bence-Jones protein, bone marrow aspiration and trephine.
Bone marrow plasma cells with abnormal morphology or composing over 20% of the nucleated cells and Bence-Jones proteinuria suggest myeloma.

C Exclude the causes of monoclonal gammopathy, such as autoimmune disease and chronic infection. Keep under review, monitoring her full blood count, ESR, immunoglobulin levels and paraprotein levels. Myeloma would be suggested by the development of anaemia, renal failure, Bence-Jones proteinuria and rising levels of paraprotein with immunoparesis.

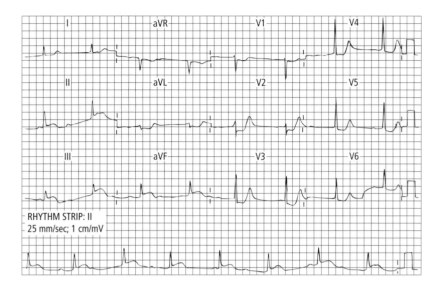

RHYTHM STRIP: II
25 mm/sec; 1 cm/mV

This 55-year-old male presented with a one-hour history of feeling unwell, sweaty and nauseated with left arm discomfort. He had a syncopal episode prior to admission. The initial blood pressure was 130/80 mmHg and his urine output was well maintained.

What is the diagnosis?

Acute infero-posterior myocardial infarction complicated by complete heart block.

There is ST elevation inferiorly with ST depression in the anterior leads. There are no Q waves in the inferior leads. The ventricular rate is 42/min whist the atrial rate is 72/min. There is atrioventricular dissociation. There is a narrow complex escape rhythm but this cannot be relied upon, particularly in the setting of acute myocardial ischaemia.

Complete heart block may occur acutely following myocardial infarction, particularly involving the inferior wall (an area with a blood supply from the right coronary artery). The atrioventricular branch of the right coronary artery also supplies the atrioventricular node and bundle of His, thus explaining this association.

A 61-year-old male was admitted via the casualty room with a two-week history of rigors and increasing jaundice. He had a past medical history of cholangiocarcinoma in the common bile duct and had previously undergone insertion of a biliary stent.

The results of his initial investigations are shown below:

Bilirubin 311 µmol/l, alkaline phosphatase 870 IU/l, AST 31 IU/l, ALT 54 IU/l, total protein 61 g/l, albumin 26 g/l, globulins 35 g/l.

CRP 181 mg/l.

Hb 11 g/dl, WCC 10×10^9/l, Plts 290×10^9/l.

A What is the most likely explanation for this man's current presentation?

B What further tests are necessary to confirm your initial impression?

C What would be your initial management?

A Blocked biliary stent with consequent ascending cholangitis and septicaemia.

B Blood cultures.
Abdominal ultrasound: this would reveal the presence of a dilated biliary duct system.
ERCP: to confirm biliary stent obstruction.

C Treatment of the septicaemia with antibiotics, e.g. ampicillin.
Ultimately, replacement of the blocked biliary stent will be the definitive treatment.

Cholangiocarcinoma may occur following infestation by liver flukes (particularly in the Far East) or on the basis of congenital hepatobiliary disease: polycystic disease of the liver or a choledochal cyst. Treatment is surgical resection (if possible) or the insertion of a biliary stent (for palliative relief of the obstructive jaundice).

This patient presented with abnormal liver function tests with an elevated alkaline phosphatase level, indicating an obstructive pathology. Jaundice and septicaemia, on the basis of biliary tree obstruction, may be the presenting features, as in this case.

An 80-year-old female was transferred to the medical admissions ward from her nursing home. She suffered from dementia and no history was available. Her nursing home letter indicated that she had a VVI pacemaker implanted 6 years previously but had been lost to follow-up for the past 3 years. She was noted to be generally unwell on the day of admission. Her pulse was noted to be 30/min. A rhythm strip of her limb leads is shown below.

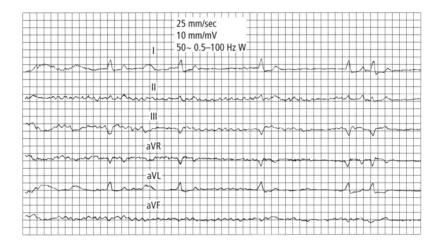

A What ECG abnormalities are illustrated?

B What further investigations are necessary to investigate the cause of the bradycardia further?

A Atrial fibrillation with a slow ventricular response.

B In the absence of any pacing spikes pacemaker failure must be suspected. Therefore pacemaker interrogation is necessary with a chest radiograph to determine lead position and integrity.

An elderly female was admitted to the orthopaedic ward having fractured her hip. She had a past history of congestive cardiac failure for which she was taking thiazide and loop diuretics. Her urea and electrolytes on admission were normal. Surgical intervention was undertaken for her fractured hip. Three days post-operatively she was drowsy and confused.

Repeat blood tests produced the following results:

Sodium 105 mmol/l, potassium 2.6 mmol/l, bicarbonate 31 mmol/l, urea 5.3 mmol/l, creatinine 80 µmol/l.

Arterial blood gases: pH 7.58, PO_2 10.7 kPa, pCO_2 4.6 kPa, base excess 12 mmol/l.

A What are the biochemical abnormalities demonstrated?

B What is the most likely cause for this?

C Name three common medical conditions in which this phenomenon may also occur.

A Hyponatraemic, hypokalaemic alkalosis.

B The over-infusion of intravenous fluids post-operatively, in addition to the use of diuretic therapy, has resulted in a dilutional hyponatraemia and hypokalaemia. The management would be to discontinue the diuretics and commence fluid restriction to correct the sodium concentration. Oral potassium supplements are also indicated.

C Dilutional hyponatraemia is also seen in nephrotic syndrome, liver cirrhosis and severe congestive cardiac failure.

Over-infusion of 5% dextrose postoperatively is a familiar cause of a dilutional hyponatraemia. The sodium losses have been aggravated in this case by the concomitant use of diuretics. Loop diuretics inhibit sodium–potassium cotransport in the ascending limb of the loop of Henle, whilst thiazides inhibit sodium transport in the distal tubule. With consequent changes in the renin–angiotensin system and antidiuretic hormone (ADH) release, the net effect is concentrated urine and fluid retention, further aggravating the hyponatraemia. Insufficient potassium supplementation has produced the dilutional hypokalaemia and subsequent alkalosis.

A woman was seen for her six-monthly review at an outpatient clinic. She had noticed increasing tiredness and a tendency to seek warm environments. A Bjork–Shiley aortic valve replacement had been fitted two years previously and her subsequent course was complicated by haemodynamically compromising ventricular tachycardia. Her medications were as follows: amiodarone, 200 mg, o.d.; frusemide/amiloride combination, 40 mg/5 mg, o.d. and warfarin.

The thyroid function tests from her visit were recorded as follows:
Free thyroxine (FT4) 8 pmol/l, TSH 18.9 mU/l, free triiodothyronine (FT3) 1.6 pmol/l.

A How would you interpret these thyroid function tests?

B What is the most likely underlying cause for this abnormality?

C What action would you recommend in the light of these tests?

A This woman shows evidence of hypothyroidism.

B This is most likely due to a drug-induced hypothyroidism consequent to her amiodarone therapy. Amiodarone has also been shown to cause hyperthyroidism, even several months following discontinuation of therapy. Amiodarone contains iodine and in addition has structural similarities to thyroxine. The mechanism by which thyroid dysfunction may occur therefore becomes clearer:
- The iodine content of the drug may influence thyroid hormone release (Wolff–Chaikoff effect).
- The peripheral metabolism of T4 to T3 is reduced resulting in a particularly low FT3.
- Occasionally iodine can cause cold nodules to warm up or patients with Graves in remission to become toxic again.

C The management of amiodarone induced hypothyroidism is simply to treat with thyroxine. Monitoring of the patient is more difficult, as the amiodarone can stimulate release of pituitary TSH by blocking the conversion of T4 to T3 within the pituitary. Thus, it is necessary to monitor the FT4 and the FT3 as well as the TSH and the clinical status of the patient. Amiodarone has a half-life of over one month, so if it is discontinued, resolution will not occur for at least six months.

A woman was referred to an on-call medical team with a history of general decline in health, malaise, nausea and muscle twitching. She had a history of ischaemic heart disease and chronic congestive cardiac failure (treated with frusemide, metolazone and captopril). Her admission 12-lead ECG is shown below.

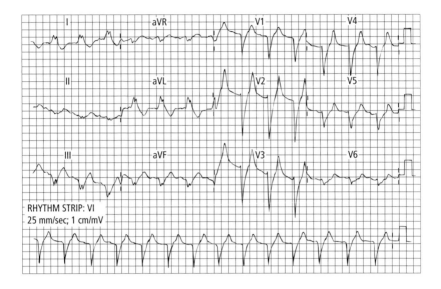

A Describe the ECG abnormalities shown.

B What is the underlying cause for these ECG changes?

C What would your immediate management of this patient be?

A Sinus rhythm, first degree heart block, left bundle branch block, tented T waves.

B Hyperkalaemia (serum potassium of 8.5 mM in this case).
The history would suggest end-stage cardiac failure with diuretic-induced acute on chronic renal failure. The uraemia is producing the muscle twitching. The ECG changes shown are the classical later changes of hyperkalaemia, the earliest changes being T-wave tenting. Later changes result in further broadening of the QRS complex with a 'sine wave' tracing and finally ventricular fibrillation and standstill may occur.

C Urgent assessment of urea and electrolytes and immediate cardiac monitoring.
Cardio-protection can be conferred immediately by administering 10 ml of 10% calcium gluconate (slow intravenous injection over 5 min). The subsequent immediate management will involve the use of the following: intravenous soluble insulin/50% dextrose regime and possibly haemodialysis (dependant on the clinical circumstances). Sodium bicarbonate (orally/intravenously) may also be used, depending on the degree of acidosis and heart failure. Intravenous salbutamol is also useful in the acute management of hyperkalaemia, although in this example its use was relatively contraindicated due to the presence of ischaemic heart disease. In the longer term, the diuretics and captopril should be discontinued and calcium resonium (orally/per rectum) commenced.

A 78-year-old male was seen in clinic with shortness of breath on exertion and peripheral oedema. He had been discharged from hospital two months earlier after a prolonged ITU stay following a respiratory arrest on the surgical ward.

Give a possible explanation for the following lung function tests:
FEV_1 0.72 l (predicted 2.21) (FEV, forced expiratory volume)
FVC 2.01 l (predicted 2.96) (FVC, forced vital capacity)
PEF 70 l/min (predicted 400) (PEF, peak expiratory flow)
TLC-He 5.65 l (predicted 5.86) (TLC-He, total lung capacity)
T_LCO 18.5 ml/min/mmHg (predicted 20.5) (T_LCO, carbon monoxide transfer factor).

Obstructive lung disease, possible tracheal stenosis.

The FEV_1/FVC ratio is 35.9% suggesting severe obstructive lung disease. However, the rest of the lung parenchymal function is essentially normal. Given his recent protracted ITU admission, this patient's problems may be secondary to tracheal stenosis following intubation.

A 50-year-old female presented with a three-month history of right upper quadrant pain that was sharp and radiated to the right shoulder. There was also a history of weight loss. Her past medical history consisted of cholecystectomy only and she was not taking any medications. On examination, she had an enlarged firm liver and a bruit was audible over the right hypochondrium. There were no stigmata of chronic liver disease.

Her initial blood investigations were as follows:

Bilirubin 12 μmol/l, alkaline phosphatase 300 IU/l, AST 50 IU/l, ALT 35 IU/l, total protein 70 g/l, albumin 36 g/l, globulins 34 g/l.

PT 14 s.

Serum alpha-fetoprotein 1200 ng/ml (normal range adult 1–10 mg/ml).

A What liver pathology would you suspect from this information?

B What is the relevance of the serum alpha-fetoprotein?

C How would you proceed to investigate this patient?

A Primary hepatocellular carcinoma.

B The alpha-fetoprotein levels may be markedly elevated in primary hepatocellular carcinoma but it must be borne in mind that elevated levels are also seen with other tumours. Germinal cell tumours of the testis and ovary and certain gastrointestinal tumours fall into this category. Levels below 1000 ng/ml may be found is severe viral hepatitis and active cirrhosis.

C Abdominal ultrasound
Liver biopsy: in particular of any echogenic lesions identified on abdominal ultrasound.

Primary hepatocellular carcinoma is relatively uncommon (in comparison to hepatic metastases) in Europe and North America. When it does occur, it tends (in the vast majority of cases) to be on a substrate of liver cirrhosis or chronic active hepatitis. The commonest aetiological factors are chronic alcoholism and hepatitis B.

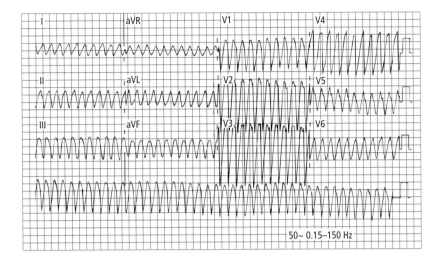

A 50-year-old male was admitted with a history of palpitations over the previous week. He had a past medical history of atrial flutter, treated by direct current cardioversion and subsequently with quinidine. He had seen his general practitioner several days prior to admission and the dose of quinidine had been increased. On this occasion, he was again found to be in atrial flutter with 2:1 block. Following a period of cardiac monitoring the medical registrar on-call was asked to review him. He had become acutely unwell with light-headedness. The blood pressure was 80/40 mmHg. An ECG was recorded and comparison with his previous ECG tracings revealed a regular broad complex tachycardia with no further widening of the QRS complexes and no axis or morphological change from previously.

A Can you comment on the ECG shown?

B What is the differential diagnosis?

A The ventricular response on the ECG shown is 260/min, having increased from the rate of 150/min which had been present when this man was in atrial flutter with 2:1 block. There is no evidence of atrioventricular dissociation.

B The differential diagnosis would be atrial flutter with 1:1 atrioventricular conduction or ventricular tachycardia. Given that the patient is haemodynamically compromised the treatment would be similar in both cases: urgent cardioversion.

Quinidine is a cinchona alkaloid and an isomer of the antimalarial, quinine. It is useful in the treatment of atrial flutter and fibrillation, although it has been recognized that it is best to control the ventricular response initially with drugs such as digoxin or beta blockers prior to the introduction of quinidine because its slowing of the atrial flutter rate and its vagolytic properties may otherwise allow 1:1 atrioventricular conduction to occur. In addition, in toxicity quinidine may promote the development of ventricular tachycardia, torsade de pointes being particularly characteristic.

A 70-year-old male presented to the medical outpatient clinic with a two-month history of anorexia, weight loss and lethargy. He had a past history of epilepsy and cerebrovascular disease, his current medications being phenytoin, aspirin and nifedipine. Clinical examination was unremarkable.

His initial blood tests were as follows:

Hb 6.6 g/dl, WCC 2.4×10^9/l, Plts 25×10^9/l, MCV 124 fl, haematocrit 0.19, MCH 43 pg, MCHC 35 g/dl, ESR 10 mm/h.

Blood film: oval macrocytes, hypersegmented neutrophils.

Liver and thyroid function tests: normal

A What are the possible causes for the pancytopenia?

B What further tests would you request?

A Vitamin B_{12} or folic acid deficiency.
Phenytoin therapy.

B Serum vitamin B_{12} and folate levels.
Reticulocyte count.
Bone marrow biopsy.
Antibodies to gastric parietal cells and intrinsic factor.
Schilling test.

A pancytopenia may occur due to decreased marrow production or increased peripheral consumption. Decreased production may be due to a megaloblastic anaemia, marrow infiltration or aplasia. Increased consumption may be seen in hypersplenism. A pancytopenia may also be seen in SLE. The presence of oval macrocytes and hypersegmented neutrophils in this case suggests the pancytopaenia is most likely to be due to the presence of a megaloblastic bone marrow, i.e. a deficiency of vitamin B_{12} or folic acid.

The commonest cause of vitamin B_{12} deficiency in Europe is pernicious anaemia, hence checking the intrinsic factor and gastric parietal cell antibody status is necessary. Deficiency of folic acid may occur with the use of anticonvulsant drugs. Indeed, phenytoin has been documented to cause a variety of haematological abnormalities, including megaloblastic anaemia, pancytopenia, aplastic anaemia, leucopenia, agranulocytosis and thrombocytopenia.

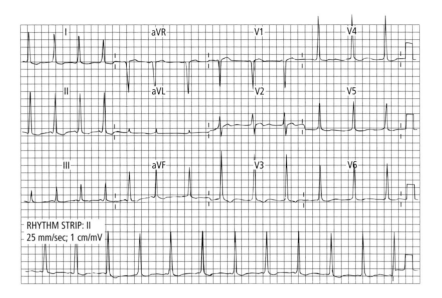

RHYTHM STRIP: II
25 mm/sec; 1 cm/mV

The ECG shown above is that of a 25-year-old female who attended casualty with recurrent and regular palpitations and dizzy spells. These had started as a child, but had worsened in severity as she had grown older. The physical examination was unremarkable. Initial investigations had shown normal thyroid function tests.

A What is the ECG diagnosis?

B Give two associations of this condition

A Wolff–Parkinson–White syndrome (short PR interval, delta wave and prolonged QRS duration best seen in lead III).

B Ebstein's anomaly.
Mitral valve prolapse.

Electrical impulses can only be conducted between the atria and ventricles via the atrioventricular node. In some individuals, however, extra connections (accessory pathways) exist, known as bypass tracts. These can occur anywhere in the atrioventricular groove, the commonest type being atrioventricular bypass tracts, which connect the atria to the ventricles. Bypass tracts may conduct anterogradely or retrogradely. Anterograde conduction in the Wolff–Parkinson–White syndrome produces the classical ECG features of a shortened PR interval (<0.12 s), prolonged QRS complex duration, due to the presence of a delta wave (a sign of pre-excitation of the ventricles due to the anterogradely conducting accessory pathway).

Traditionally, Wolff–Parkinson–White syndrome is classified as having an accessory pathway (bundle of Kent) between the left atrium and the left ventricle (type A) or between the right atrium and the right ventricle (type B). The delta wave may be biphasic or negative in leads V1–V3 (and positive in lead I) in type B, whilst it is positive in leads V1–V6 (and negative in lead I) in type A. It is, however, more useful to consider atrioventricular bypass tracts as having one of four possible locations: left or right free wall and anterior or posterior septum. The location can be defined precisely by studying the surface ECG and intracardiac mapping as part of an electrophysiological study.

Retrogradely conducting accessory pathways will not reveal their presence with the characteristic ECG changes of anterogradely conducting pathways. They are therefore said to be 'concealed' accessory pathways. Their presence may lead to the establishment of a circus rhythm with anterograde conduction along the normal atrioventricular pathway and retrograde conduction along the bypass tract resulting in macro-re-entrant atrioventricular tachycardia (AVRT).

A 40-year-old male was admitted with a history of a sore throat and dysphagia over the course of three days. He had deteriorated on the day of admission with a fever, increased vomiting and weakness. His previous history was one of Cushing's disease and this had been surgically treated 15 years ago. He was taking hydrocortisone and fludrocortisone on admission. On examination, he was febrile, with inflamed tonsils. He was deeply pigmented all over his body with a blood pressure of 100/70 mmHg. Abdominal scars were noted but physical examination was otherwise unremarkable.

His initial investigations are outlined below:

Hb 14 g/dl, WCC 19×10⁹/l, ESR 41 mm/h.

Urinalysis: ketones +++

Sodium 130 mmol/l, potassium 5.6 mmol/l, urea 5.3 mmol/l, creatinine 120 μmol/l.

A What is the diagnosis?

B What is the immediate management?

A Addisonian crisis in a patient with iatrogenic primary hypoadrenalism.

B Intravenous steroid therapy and treatment of the acute tonsillitis with intravenous antibiotics.

The treatment of Cushing's disease by bilateral total adrenalectomy is rarely practised. Its aftermath, in 10% of cases, was Nelson's syndrome: the hypersecretion of ACTH from a pituitary adenoma with the development of skin pigmentation (Addison's disease may also result in skin and mucosal pigmentation). Such patients have to be maintained on life-long steroid and mineralocorticoid replacement therapy. In the presence of an intercurrent illness, acute tonsillitis in this case, patients are normally advised to double their steroid intake. Failing this, Addisonian crisis may occur with nausea, vomiting, hypotension and hyponatraemia, as above.

The following blood results were found on a private medical screen for a 46-year-old executive:
sodium 134 mmol/l, potassium 4.4 mmol/l, urea 5.0 mmol/l, creatinine 90 µmol/l, bilirubin 34 µmol/l, AST 28 IU/l, ALT 25 IU/l, alkaline phosphatase 60 IU/l.
Hb 12.8 g/dl, Plts 254×10^9/l, WCC 5.5×10^9/l, MCV 85 fl.
Urine dipstick: N.A.D.

A What is the likeliest cause of this patient's abnormal blood results?

B What treatment is necessary?

A Gilbert's syndrome.
Named after Gilbert (1901) who described familial hyperbilirubinaemia in the absence of apparent liver disease. Although half the cases have slightly diminished red cell survival, the main mechanism is thought to be due to reduced activity of hepatic uridyldiphosphate glucuronyl transferase (UDPGT), i.e. the primary defect is one of glucuronidation (compared with Rotor and Dubin–Johnson syndromes where the major defect is in conjugation).

The differential diagnosis includes Dubin–Johnson, Rotor and Crigler–Najjar type II syndromes: the liver function tests are normal in all of these except for an elevated bilirubin level. However, they are all far less common than Gilbert's syndrome (incidence of 2–5% of the population) and are more likely to be symptomatic. In Dubin–Johnson and Rotor syndromes the bilirubin is conjugated, thereby resulting in dark urine. Crigler–Najjar syndrome is associated with a far greater reduction in UDPGT activity and in many ways is thought of as a homozygously expressed form of Gilbert's syndrome, although the liver histology in this condition is normal whereas in Gilbert's there is said to be an increase in centrilobular lipofuscin.

The bilirubin level in Gilbert's is rarely high enough to cause icterus but may rise sufficiently during nutritional compromise, as occurs in starvation or reduction in appetite due to intercurrent illness. Indeed this forms the basis of the diagnostic test for this condition, i.e. fasting looking for a doubling of the bilirubin. Alternatively, intravenous nicotinic acid produces the same effect.

B No treatment is necessary for Gilbert's syndrome.

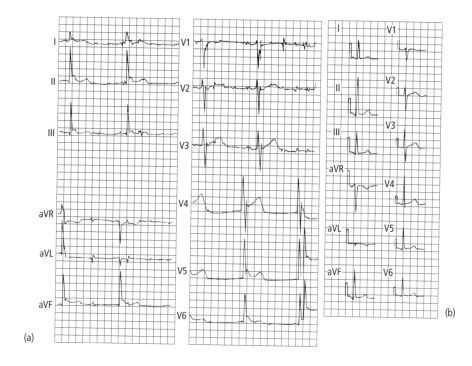

(a)

(b)

The ECGs shown above were taken of a patient before (a) and after (b) treatment.

What treatment was given to this patient?

Re-warming of the patient.

The ECG recorded before treatment (a) shows the typical changes of hypothermia: bradycardia, J waves (at the ends of the QRS complexes) and shivering artefacts. These changes reverse (as seen in b) on re-warming.

The medical registrar was asked to review an elderly patient on the surgical wards who had a potassium level of 7.0 mmol/l.

The results of subsequent investigations are shown:

Plasma: sodium 130 mmol/l, potassium 7.0 mmol/l, urea 30 mmol/l, creatinine 240 µmol/l, osmolality 294 mosmol/l

Urine: sodium 5 mmol/l, urea 350 mmol/l, osmolality 450 mosmol/l

A What is the probable cause of the results presented above?

B What would be your initial line of management?

A Acute renal failure due to inadequate post-operative hydration and tubulo-interstitial disease.

Acute renal failure may be divided up into pre-renal (e.g. intravascular volume depletion due to dehydration or blood loss), renal parenchymal (e.g. glomerulonephritis, interstitial or tubular nephritis) and postrenal causes (e.g. renal stones or prostatic hypertrophy).

Pre-renal and renal parenchymal disorders can be diagnosed based on spot urine and plasma data, assuming that the patient has not been given diuretics.

Pre-renal renal failure
　Spot urine: Na < 20 mmol/l,
　Urinary urea: plasma urea > 20:1,
　Urinary osmolality: plasma osmolality > 1.5:1.
Renal parenchymal dysfunction
　Spot urine: Na > 20 mmol/l,
　Urinary urea: plasma urea < 10:1,
　Urine osmolality: plasma osmolality < 1.5:1,
　Active urinary sediment may be present.

B The initial management should concentrate on reducing the potassium level, and then controlling the renal failure:

- Insertion of a central venous catheter and appropriate fluid replacement to a central venous pressure of 9–13 cmH$_2$O. This, *per se*, will usually result in an improvement in the serum potassium level;
- Urinary catheterization to determine accurate urinary output: if oliguric, cautious rehydration is advised;
- If the hyperkalaemia persists in spite of rehydration, an insulin in dextrose infusion may be administered;
- Calcium gluconate given as an intravenous bolus to stabilize the myocardium.

A 36-year-old female is on treatment for primary biliary cirrhosis (PBC). Her full blood count is shown below:
Hb 11.5 g/dl, WCC 6.5×10⁹/l, Plts 205×10⁹/l, MCV 104 fl.

Give the three likeliest causes of the blood abnormality presented above.

Liver dysfunction secondary to cirrhosis.
Associated autoimmune hypothyroidism.
Cytotoxic agent therapy.

PBC is associated with a variety of autoimmune and nonautoimmune conditions, as shown below:
- Sjögren's syndrome
- Systemic sclerosis
- CREST syndrome
- Autoimmune hypothyroidism
- Renal tubular acidosis
- Coeliac disease
- Dermatomyositis

    Treatment for this condition involves replacement of fat soluble vitamins (A,D,E and K), cholestyramine (for the pruritis) and disease-modifying agents. The latter includes steroids, which improve the liver histology (as does D-penicillamine) but are relatively contraindicated due to their deleterious effects on vitamin D deficient bone in this condition. Azathioprine is said to be of partial benefit and newer agents include methotrexate, colchicine, and ursodiol. The definitive treatment remains liver transplantation.

    Causes of macrocytosis include: Vitamin B_{12} and folate deficiency, reticulocytosis, alcohol, liver disease, hypopituitarism and hypothyroidism, myelodysplasia, multiple myeloma, acquired sideroblastic anaemia, aplastic anaemia, cytotoxic drug therapy, phenytoin, pregnancy and Down's syndrome.

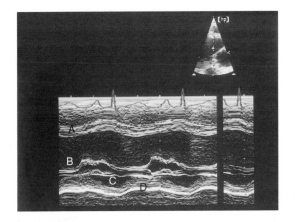

A 38-year-old female presented with shortness of breath on exertion. There is a childhood history of scarlet fever. There is a loud first heart sound and mid-diastolic murmur present.

A What is this investigation?

B Name structures A to D on the diagram

C What is the likely underlying diagnosis?

A Transthoracic echocardiogram (M-mode recording).

B

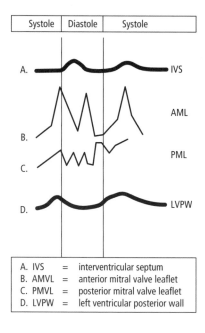

Systole	Diastole	Systole

A. — IVS

AML

B.

PML

C.

D. — LVPW

A. IVS	=	interventricular septum
B. AMVL	=	anterior mitral valve leaflet
C. PMVL	=	posterior mitral valve leaflet
D. LVPW	=	left ventricular posterior wall

C Mild mitral stenosis.

This echocardiogram shows thickened calcified mitral valve leaflets. The classic M shape of the mitral valve is still preserved: the first diastolic peak is due to passive filling of the left ventricle and the second peak due to active filling in late diastole secondary to atrial contraction. As the degree of mitral stenosis worsens, the excursion of the two leaflets is reduced as the posterior mitral valve leaflet moves anteriorly with the anterior leaflet. The anterior leaflet excursion and the slope of mitral valve closure are reduced in this case; the latter becomes horizontal in severe stenosis. The second AMVL peak (due to atrial contraction) is often lost in moderate-severe mitral stenosis with the onset of atrial fibrillation.

An 18-year-old, educationally subnormal female was brought to an outpatient clinic by her foster parents. They were concerned about her small stature. She had been seen previously for several behavioural problems including self-harm and recurrent bed-wetting. The patient was normotensive.

The following blood and urine results were noted:

Plasma: Sodium 138 mmol/l, potassium 2.5 mmol/l, urea 4.0 mmol/l, creatinine 90 μmol/l.

Urine: increased potassium and chloride excretion.

Blood gases on air: pH 7.5, pCO_2 4.5 kPa, pO_2 12.5 kPa, HCO_3 34 mmol/l.

A What is the likely underlying diagnosis in this girl's case?
Give a differential diagnosis.

B How would you treat this patient?

A Bartter's syndrome.

The differential in this case includes:

Laxative abuse/ Diuretic abuse/ Liquorice overdose/ Bulimia.

The diagnosis of Bartter's syndrome is suggested by the constellation of syndromic features, including low IQ and small stature. However, one should consider the other possibilities outlined above, which may be differentiated biochemically by analysis of urinary potassium and chloride excretion as described below.

Bartter first described the syndrome in 1962 as hyperreninism from juxtaglomerular hypertrophy which may also have the associated features of small stature, impaired IQ, weakness, and nocturnal enuresis, thought to be secondary to potassium depletion nephropathy. The blood pressure is normal due to intravascular volume depletion.

It has a familial tendency and is often diagnosed in childhood. The patient may, however, present much later in their late teens or early twenties. The typical biochemical picture is of hypokalaemic, hypochloraemic metabolic alkalosis with raised urinary potassium and chloride excretion. The mechanism is thought to involve defective chloride resorption in the ascending loop of Henle leading to sodium and water loss. This, in turn, causes an increase in renin and aldosterone secretion.

The differential diagnosis of hypokalaemic metabolic alkalosis with normal blood pressure is discussed below:

- Diuretic abuse: initially associated with a rise in urinary chloride excretion that subsequently falls.
- Laxative abuse: obviously associated with diarrhoea. Although the urinary chloride excretion is said to be low, the urinary potassium excretion can be high in the event of a severe metabolic alkalosis or if the potassium depletion is extreme.
- Bulimia: associated with a low urinary chloride.
- Villous adenoma: diarrhoea with low urinary potassium.
- Primary renal tubular disorder, e.g. cystinosis or renal tubular acidosis.
- Chronic pyloric stenosis.
- Liquorice overdose.

B Recognized treatments for this condition include the use of indomethacin as a first line agent along with potassium replacement therapy. One could also consider the use of potassium sparing diuretics, e.g. amiloride and triamterene. ACE inhibitors are said to cause a profound drop in blood pressure.

A 65-year-old male presented to the outpatient clinic with a three-year history of back pain.

The following tests were performed:

sodium 135 mmol/l, potassium 4.5 mmol/l, urea 7.0 mmol/l, creatinine 120 µmol/l, albumin 40 g/l, total protein 60 g/l, calcium 2.4 mmol/l, phosphate 0.97 mmol/l.

Hb 14.5 g/dl, WCC 7.0×10⁹/l, Plts 220×10⁹/l.

Marrow aspirate: <10% plasma cells seen.

Urine dipstick: protein +.

A What is the likeliest cause of this man's back problems?

B Give three points to support your answer.

C Does the result of the urine dipstick help in this case?

A Osteoporosis.

B The likeliest cause of back pain in a man of this age with a history of this length would be degenerative bone disease. The extremely long history points against a diagnosis of myeloma. Other features which would make myeloma unlikely are: less than 10% plasma cells in the bone marrow aspirate; paraprotein less than 20 g/dl for an IgG paraproteinaemia and less than 10 g/dl for an IgA or IgM paraproteinaemia; normal renal function and serum calcium.

C No, this can be normal. Bence-Jones proteins are not detectable on dipstick.

A 63-year-old male was admitted with bilateral pleural effusions. A battery of tests was conducted including the following thyroid function tests (normal range in brackets):
thyroxine 78 nmol/l (58–174), free T4 14.7 pmol/l (13–30), TSH 7.80 mU/l (0.3–6.0)

A What is this patient's thyroid status?

B How would you treat his pleural effusions?

A Subclinical hypothyroidism, with normal free thyroxine but elevated TSH. It is worth checking for antithyroid antibodies. If they are positive, or the TSH rises to > 8 mU/l, then it is worth treating with thyroxine. When doing so, one should aim to normalize the TSH.

B Pleural aspiration if significant respiratory distress. The aspirate should be analysed for protein, glucose and cellular content, to exclude malignancy as a cause. A chest radiograph or CT scan of the chest should be carried out postdrainage for the same reason. The pleural effusions are unlikely to have anything to do with the subclinical hypothyroidism.

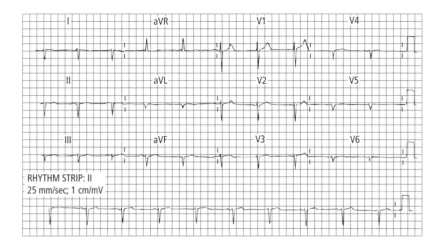

RHYTHM STRIP: II
25 mm/sec; 1 cm/mV

A 27-year-old male was referred to a medical outpatient clinic with a history of shortness of breath. His past medical history included recurrent sinus and chest infections. Clinical examination revealed early finger clubbing with bibasal pulmonary crepitations. The heart sounds were distant and not clearly defined. His 12-lead ECG is shown above.

A What ECG abnormalities are evident?

B What is the diagnosis?

C What are the other possible associated features of this condition?

A R wave progression reversed (R waves increase in size from V6 to V1) and right axis deviation. This appearance is consistent with presence of dextrocardia.

B Kartagener's syndrome.

C Kartagener's syndrome is the association of sinusitis, bronchiectasis, dextrocardia and male infertility. In some cases situs inversus may also occur. It has an autosomal recessive inheritance.

A 32-year-old male was seen in casualty with headache, lethargy, nausea and vomiting. He had a two-week history of night sweats, and had been HIV positive for two years. He had a past medical history of intraoral and gastric Kaposi's sarcoma, oesophageal candidiasis and cryptococcal meningitis a year earlier, for which he was taking prophylactic fluconazole. He was also on dapsone, rifabutin, and omeprazole.

On examination, he was pyrexial at 37.2°C, and had obvious gingival and palatal Kaposi's lesions. The remainder of the clinical examination was unremarkable and he was Kernig's sign negative, with a normal mental test score.

The results of his tests are shown:

Hb 6.8 g/dl, WCC 2.3×10^9/l, Plts 187×10^9/l.

Sodium 134 mmol/l, potassium 4.3 mmol/l, urea 9.0 mmol/l, creatinine 78 μmol/l, glucose 5.5 mmol/l.

Serum cryptococcal antigen positive.

MRI brain: no abnormality seen.

CSF: 2 lymphocytes, 1 red blood cell; protein 0.24 g/dl, glucose 2.7 mmol/l.

A What further tests would you request on the CSF?

B What is the likely differential diagnosis?

A India ink stain.
Ziehl-Nielsen.

B Cryptococcal meningitis/tuberculous meningitis.

The history of headache and pyrexia of indolent course is typical of cryptococcal meningitis. Relapse of this illness, despite prophylaxis, is also common, as in this case. The CSF findings are nonspecific in this illness, and the normal protein and relatively normal cell count in this case should not detract from making the diagnosis, although the serum cryptococcal antigen test must be positive. The MRI scan can often be normal, but can show a speckled appearance due to the presence of cryptococcomata. Treatment is with amphotericin B and fluconazole, although fluconazole, in full rather than prophylactic dose, alone is being used. Prophylaxis with life-long fluconazole is then recommended.

Tuberculous meningitis should be considered but is less likely given the normal CSF lymphocyte and protein levels. Toxoplasmosis is unlikely with the normal MRI scan. CMV and HSV encephalitis are unlikely given the indolent course and the normal conscious level in this case.

A 60-year-old male presented with a history of increasing exertional dyspnoea, orthopnoea and paroxysmal nocturnal dyspnoea. He had a past history of an atrial septal defect repair 20 years previously with documented mitral valve prolapse. More recently, he had hypertension and ischaemic heart disease diagnosed. On examination, he was in controlled atrial fibrillation and had a pansystolic murmur with congestive cardiac failure.

His cardiac catheterization data were as follows:

Pressure measurements (mmHg): Right atrial mean 12; Right ventricle 38/5; Pulmonary artery 40/14 (mean pressure 24); Pulmonary capillary wedge pressure mean 14, v wave 20; Left ventricle 159/9; Aorta 145/60; Mitral valve gradient 6.

Right ventricular angiography: no tricuspid incompetence.

Oxygen saturation measurements (%): Superior vena cava 59, Inferior vena cava 71, High right atrium 60, Mid-right atrium 64, Lower right atrium 66, Right ventricular apex 62, Left ventricle 95.

A What is the likely cause of the pansystolic murmur?

B Is there a left to right shunt present?

A Mitral incompetence — this would be clearly seen on left ventricular angiography.

B The oxygen saturation data do not demonstrate the presence of a significant left to right shunt.

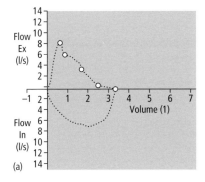

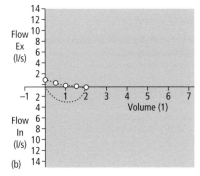

The flow-volume loop to the right (b) is that of a 78-year-old male weighing 81 kg and 162 cm tall. What comments would you make about this loop, as compared to the normal flow-volume loop, for a male weighing 105 kg and 180 cm tall, shown on the left (a).

Severe obstructive defect, as in asthma or chronic obstructive airways disease.
Reduced lung volume.

The flow-volume loop shows very poor expiratory flow with better (but not normal) inspiratory flow in keeping with asthma.

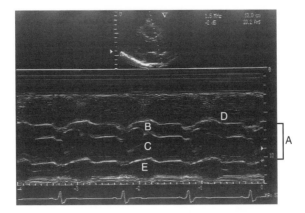

This 30-year-old male was noted to have a heart murmur as part of an occupational health screening examination. There was no past history of note. A transthoracic echocardiogram was undertaken.

Name structures A–C in this M-mode recording.
What is the cause of the murmur?

A diagrammatic representation of a normal M-mode recording taken across the aortic root in the parasternal long axis view is shown below. The closure line of the aortic valve leaflets is shown positioned in the centre of the aortic root. The M-mode echocardiographic recording shown is that of a bicuspid aortic valve where the closure line of the valve is eccentric. Doming of the leaflets may be seen in systole. There is an association with coarctation of the aorta.

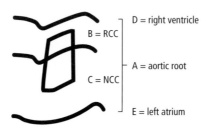

D = right ventricle

B = RCC

A = aortic root

C = NCC

E = left atrium

RCC = right coronary cusp of aortic valve
NCC = non-coronary cusp

A 17-year-old anorexic patient, who was severely malnourished, was being parenterally fed. The psychiatrists asked for a medical opinion on receiving the following blood test results:

Hb 12.9 g/dl, WCC 2.68×10^9/l, Plts 77×10^9/l.

Sodium 139 mmol/l, potassium 4.0 mmol/l, bicarbonate 26.5 mmol/l, urea 10.9 mmol/l, creatinine 76 µmol/l, albumin 34 g/l, alkaline phosphatase 597 IU/l, ALT 66 IU/l, bilirubin 21 µmol/l, calcium 2.0 mmol/l, phosphate 0.78 mmol/l.

How would you explain the above results?

Anorexia, *per se*, has been associated with a variety of metabolic and haematological abnormalities. Pancytopenia and leukopenia are seen with a bone marrow showing marrow hypoplasia, absence of fat cells and infiltration with mature lymphocytes; these changes are treatable with recombinant human colony stimulating factor. If the patient has reached the stage of severe malnourishment then multiorgan failure can result. The patient's cholestatic liver function picture is probably secondary to the parenteral nutrition.

The raised alkaline phosphatase may be due to vitamin D deficiency, osteomalacia and secondary hypothyroidism. Thus alkaline phosphatase isoenzymes (bone versus liver) and vitamin D/PTH levels should be checked.

A 63-year-old female was referred to a medical outpatient clinic. She was largely symptomless but due to feelings of general lethargy her general practitioner had requested several blood tests, the results of which had precipitated her referral (see below). She denied significant alcohol consumption and was a vegan. Her past history was that until the menopause she had suffered from menorrhagia and had recently been found to be in atrial fibrillation (taking digoxin). Her uncle, an alcoholic, had diagnosed chronic liver disease. Clinical examination was unremarkable, although atrial fibrillation was confirmed.

Her initial investigations were reported as follows:

Bilirubin 12 µmol/l, alkaline phosphatase 90 IU/l, AST 40 IU/l, ALT 35 IU/l, total protein 70 g/l, albumin 37 g/l, globulin 33 g/l.

Hb 14 g/dl, WCC 4×10⁹/l, Plts 170×10⁹/l, MCV 99 fl, serum iron 31 µmol/l, transferrin 2.5 g/l, ferritin 700 ng/ml.

A What is the likely diagnosis?

B What further confirmatory test is required and what result would you anticipate?

C How would you manage this patient?

A Hereditary haemochromatosis (HHC).

B Elevated fasting early morning transferrin saturation. Genetic testing for mutations within HFE gene. Up to 93% of patients with suspected HHC are homozygous for the C282Y point mutation.

In selected cases, liver biopsy may still be required. This shows increased iron storage within the hepatocytes (Perls' Prussian blue stain) with subsequent development of hepatic fibrosis and cirrhosis.

C This woman has avoided significant iron overload previously due to her diet and menorrhagia. She will now require regular venesection in order to prevent iron overload.

This inherited condition results from an abnormal deposition of excess iron stores within various organs, e.g. the liver, heart and pancreas producing organ dysfunction as a consequence. Classically, the patient will present with 'bronze diabetes' (due to damage to the pancreatic islets and increased skin pigmentation) and hepatomegaly. Heart involvement may produce cardiac arrhythmias and cardiac failure. Hypogonadism and arthritis are related features.

A 60-year-old male has a history of syncopal episodes. His 12-lead ECG is shown below.

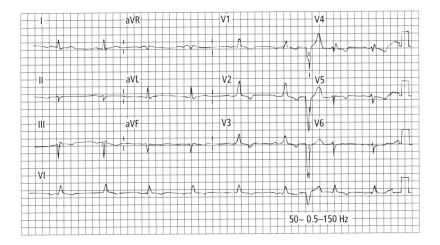

50~ 0.5–150 Hz

A Describe the ECG abnormalities shown.

B What further investigation is necessary?

A Sinus rhythm, ventricular ectopic beat, right bundle branch block in the presence of left axis deviation (left anterior hemi-block), bifid P waves.

B 24-h tape.

A 46-year-old epileptic male was admitted in status epilepticus. His epileptic control had been deteriorating recently and his regular antiepileptic agent had been increased by his general practitioner. He was noted to have lobar pneumonia and was treated on high dose intravenous benzylpenicillin.

His blood results prior to treatment are shown below:

Hb 9.6 g/dl, WCC 5.1 × 10^9/l, Plts 48 × 10^9/l, PT 18 s, APTT 41 s.

Sodium 136 mmol/l, potassium 3.4 mmol/l, urea 8.0 mmol/l, creatinine 152 µmol/l.

Explain the blood results presented above.

The cause of this patient's problems is probably his antiepileptic medication, which had been recently increased. High levels of sodium valproate can cause reversible prolongation of bleeding time and a decrease in platelets. Red cell hypoplasia and leucopenia are rarely reported.

A 26-year-old male returned from a trip to the Rajastan area of India with pyrexia, rigors, headache and malaise.

A blood test revealed the following results:

Hb 15.2 g/dl, WCC 6.0×10^9/l, Plts 90×10^9/l.

Blood film: Ring forms of *Plasmodium falciparum* seen (2.2% parasitaemia).

He was started on intravenous quinine and initially made good progress, but was found unrousable the next morning.

What is the likely cause of this man's sudden demise?

Probable hypoglycaemic coma precipitated by intravenous quinine: it is imperative to monitor the blood glucose when using this agent and some advocate a 10% dextrose drip running throughout its infusion. Hypoglycaemia can also occur in falciparum malaria in the absence of quinine therapy. Cerebral malaria is also a possibility, especially given the prevalence of malignant falciparum malaria in Rajastan. This condition is caused by the sludging of red blood cells in the cerebral capillaries and presents as a gradual decline in conscious level, often with fitting preceding coma.

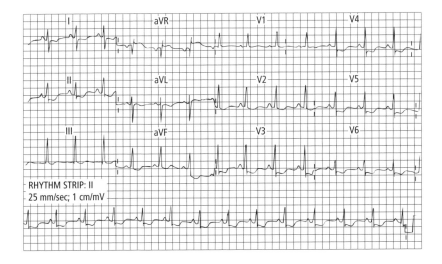

A 27-year-old female was referred to a general medical clinic with a history of exertional dyspnoea which had been increasing over the previous six months. She had a past medical history of childhood asthma and was a smoker. Her only regular medication was the oral contraceptive pill. The chest radiograph was normal. Her 12-lead ECG is shown.

A Describe the ECG abnormalities demonstrated.

B What is the most likely diagnosis?

C What is the aetiology?

A P pulmonale, right axis deviation, right ventricular hypertrophy with right ventricular strain pattern.

B Pulmonary hypertension, primary or secondary.

C Pulmonary thrombo-embolic disease consequent to the use of the oral contraceptive pill will need to be excluded.

A 52-year-old male with *Pneumocystis carinii* (PCP) pneumonia and AIDS had a *grand mal* fit on the ward. The following blood and arterial gas results were noted:

Sodium 113 mmol/l, potassium 5.2 mmol/l, urea 8.6 mmol/l, creatinine 76 µmol/l.

Arterial blood gases on 40% inspired oxygen: pH 7.45, pCO_2 4.11 kPa, pO_2 6.15 kPa, standard bicarbonate 24.1 mmol/l, oxygen saturation 86%.

A What are the possible causes of his fit in this context?

B What is the differential diagnosis for his hyponatraemia?

A Hypoxia.
Hyponatraemia.
Space occupying lesion, e.g. cerebral toxoplasmosis, lymphoma, cerebral abscess.
Progressive multifocal leucoencephalopathy.
Encephalitis, e.g. herpes simplex, cytomegalovirus.

B Syndrome of inappropriate antidiuretic hormone secretion (SIADH).
Adrenal insufficiency.
Secondary to cotrimoxazole.
Ketoconazole treatment.

SIADH is the commonest cause of hyponatraemia in the setting of HIV in many studies. Chest infection with PCP could also be a precipitant of SIADH in this case. Adrenalitis is a common finding at postmortem in AIDS, with cytomegalovirus (CMV) being the commonest cause. Other causes of adrenalitis include toxoplasmosis, *Cryptococcus*, *Mycobacterium tuberculosis*, *Mycobacterium avium intracellulare*, Kaposi's sarcoma, lymphoma and even direct HIV infection of the adrenals. Co-trimoxazole, used in the treatment of PCP, can also cause hyporeninaemic hypoaldosteronism, and ketoconazole, used as an antifungal agent causes a drop in cortisol and aldosterone levels.

A 50-year-old male had been diagnosed as having aortic stenosis with normal coronary arteries one year previously and underwent aortic valve replacement (Bjork–Shiley prosthesis). The pre-operative echocardiogram had demonstrated good left ventricular function. He presented with increasing exertional dyspnoea. On examination, normal prosthetic valve sounds were audible with a soft early diastolic murmur.

His cardiac catheterization data were as follows:

Pressure measurements (mmHg): Right atrium a wave 10, v wave 10, mean 8; Right ventricle 36/8; Pulmonary artery 30/24; Pulmonary capillary wedge pressure mean 27, Aorta 140/75.

A How would you interpret the available pressure data with respect to prosthetic valve function?

B What additional investigation would most aid in the further evaluation of this patient?

A Although he had reasonable left ventricular function preoperatively, the high pulmonary capillary wedge pressure shows high left atrial pressures in this patient. This may be indicative of a high left ventricular end diastolic pressure (suggesting impaired left ventricular function or left ventricular volume overload) or may indicate prosthetic valve dysfunction (causing left ventricular volume overload).

B Transoesophageal echocardiography; this would allow detailed assessment of the aortic valve replacement, particularly in the detection of paravalvular leaks. In addition, it would allow the assessment of left ventricular function.

What is the likely pathological diagnosis based on the lung function tests of this 72-year-old male, who is cyanosed and clubbed?

FEV_1 2.00 l (predicted 2.61) (FEV, forced expiratory volume)

FVC 2.04 l (predicted 3.55) (FVC, forced vital capacity)

TLC-He 3.99 l (predicted 6.82) (TLC-He, total lung capacity)

T_LCO 1.68 ml/min/mmHg (predicted 4.58) (T_LCO, carbon monoxide transfer factor)

(TLC-He, the total lung capacity as measured by helium; T_LCO, the transfer factor for carbon monoxide.)

Fibrosing alveolitis.

The FEV_1/FVC is 97.9% suggestive of a restrictive disorder. The very low T_LCO is supportive of pathology at the alveolar membrane. Together with the history of cyanosis and clubbing, the likely diagnosis is fibrosing alveolitis.

There are two categories of lung disease, differentiated by lung function tests:

Obstructive	Restrictive
FEV_1/FVC < 75%	FEV_1/FVC > 75%
↑ RV	↓ RV, VC, TLC
↑↑ RV/TLC	↑ RV/TLC
(RV, residual volume)	

A 16-year-old female was admitted with a one-week history of sore throat, dysphagia and malaise. She had been given antibiotics by her general practitioner and had developed an itchy rash over her trunk. On examination, she was apyrexial with enlarged cervical lymph nodes. Abdominal examination revealed two-finger-breadth hepatomegaly and a palpable splenic tip. A maculopapular rash was present over her trunk and chest.

The following results were recorded:

Urea & electrolytes: normal.

Bilirubin 24 μmol/l, albumin 31 g/l, alkaline phosphatase 165 IU/l, ALT 479 IU/l.

Hb 12.5 g/dl, W.C.C 8.5 × 10^9/l, Plts 142 × 10^9/l.

What is the likely differential diagnosis?

Infectious mononucleosis (Epstein–Barr virus infection)/ Hepatitis A,B or C/ Toxoplasmosis/ HIV seroconversion reaction.

   The differential of the clinical picture presented above includes a variety of mainly viral infections. The likeliest cause in a patient of this age with no travel history or risks for HIV is glandular fever. The rash may be as a result of the infection or in response to the antibiotics given (presumably amoxycillin).

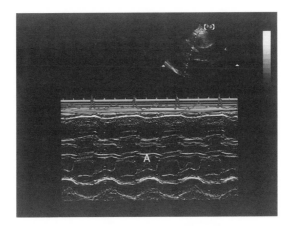

A 50-year-old female is referred with a history of exertional dyspnoea, chest pain and presyncope. On examination there is an audible ejection systolic murmur.

A What is the term applied to process A in the above M-mode echocardiograph?

B What is the likely underlying diagnosis?

A Systolic anterior motion of mitral valve apparatus (SAM).

B Hypertrophic cardiomyopathy

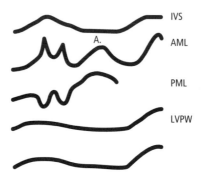

This example shows the presence of SAM: the movement of the tip of the anterior mitral valve leaflet into the left ventricular outflow tract during systole. Thickening of the tip of the anterior mitral valve leaflet may also be seen. A dynamic gradient may occur within the left ventricular outflow tract and premature closure of the aortic valve is seen.

A renal transplant patient on azathioprine was seen for follow up in an outpatient clinic. The patient had recently seen his general practitioner for painful swelling of the finger joints on his right hand and had been started on appropriate treatment.

His current full blood count compared to the previous months is shown:

Current: Hb 5.5 g/dl, Plts 30×10^9/l, WCC 2.5×10^9/l.

Previous month: Hb 9.8 g/dl, Plts 170×10^9/l, WCC 5.5×10^9/l.

Give a likely explanation for the change in full blood count.

The patient has been given allopurinol for probable gout. Allopurinol inhibits xanthine oxidase, which converts azathioprine active metabolites into inactive 6-thiouric acid. The build-up of active metabolites causes bone marrow suppression; it is generally recommended that when allopurinol is used together with azathioprine, the dose of azathioprine should be reduced by at least a quarter.

A 45-year-old male was admitted to casualty with severe central chest pain. He had been seen in a cardiology outpatient clinic two weeks earlier following a positive exercise test. His fasting cholesterol in clinic was noted to be high and he was started on appropriate treatment. The physical examination and ECG in casualty were both unremarkable. The cardiac enzyme results were CPK 900 IU/l and AST 120 IU/l.

A What is the likeliest cause of this man's chest pain?

B How would you treat him?

A This patient was started on simvastatin for his elevated cholesterol. Drugs of this class are associated with a myopathy in <0.1% of patients and the muscle tenderness so produced can lead to severe pain, as in this case. The creatinine kinase levels should be at least 10 or more times greater than normal if this diagnosis is to be entertained.

B Stop the simvastatin and give pain relief.

A 40-year-old male was referred to a medical outpatient clinic with a history of dizziness and syncope related to exertion. There was an ejection systolic murmur audible on clinical examination.

At cardiac catheterization the following information was obtained:

Pressure measurements (mmHg): Right atrium mean 4; Right ventricle 30/6; Pulmonary artery 26/10, mean 18; Pulmonary artery wedge pressure mean 8; Left ventricle 242/12; Aorta 190/95.

Left ventriculogram: good systolic function, left ventricular hypertrophy.

Coronary angiography: normal.

A What is the diagnosis?

B What is the classical triad of symptoms with which this condition may present?

C What additional investigation is necessary?

A Moderate aortic stenosis.

B Exertional presyncope/syncope, chest pain and dyspnoea.

C A recent transthoracic echocardiogram will be essential. This will help to exclude rheumatic involvement of other heart valves (particularly the mitral valve), provide corroboration of the aortic valve gradient and provide a detailed morphological assessment of the aortic valve. The latter can be useful in differentiating between a rheumatic aetiology, degenerative calcific aortic stenosis and a bicuspid aortic valve. It can exclude left ventricular outflow tract obstruction, e.g. a subaortic membrane. It will also document the presence of left ventricular hypertrophy.

A 46-year-old female was referred to a outpatient clinic with a two-month history of wheeze and cough productive of yellow sputum. She had been prescribed two courses of antibiotics and bronchodilatory inhalers, without significant benefit. A diuretic agent had recently been given for shortness of breath and pulmonary crepitations on auscultation. In clinic she complained of a persistent nasal drip, and had a left-sided foot drop.

Investigations gave the following results:

Hb 11.1 g/dl, Plts 299×10⁹/l, WCC 9.7×10⁹/l, (neutrophils 5.0, lymphocytes 1.3, monocytes 0.5, eosinophils 2.8, basophils 0.1), ESR 70 mm/h.

Sodium 139 mmol/l, potassium 5.8 mmol/l, urea 22.8 mmol/l, creatinine 303 μmol/l.

A What is the unifying diagnosis?

B What further tests would you perform to confirm this?

A Churg–Strauss syndrome.

B Renal biopsy.

This patient has a combination of asthmatic symptoms, eosinophilia, an elevated erythrocyte sedimentation rate and renal impairment: a constellation very suggestive of Churg–Stauss syndrome. This medium vessel granulomatous vasculitis has a male preponderance peaking in the fourth decade. It presents with asthma, eosinophilia of greater than 1.5 and vasculitis. Other signs include a rash (which may be maculopapular, utricarial or purpuric), abdominal pain, mononeuritis multiplex and a focal segmental glomerulonephritis. It is usually very amenable to steroid treatment.

A 42-year-old Australian female presented to casualty with fever. She had not passed urine for the entire day. She gave a past medical history of chronic back pain and had moved to the UK two months earlier. Examination was unremarkable.

Investigations gave the following results:

Sodium 132 mmol/l, potassium 5.0 mmol/l, urea 20 mmol/l, creatinine 330 µmol/l, bicarbonate 22 mmol/l, Albumin 38 g/l, total protein 55 g/l.

Serum electrophoresis normal.

Hb 12.5 g/dl, Plts 250 × 10⁹/l, WCC 7.2 × 10⁹/l, (neutrophils 3.8, lymphocytes 1.5, eosinophils 1.3, monocytes 0.5, basophils 0.1), ESR 50 mm/h.

Lumbar spine radiograph: osteoarthritic change only.

A What is the underlying cause of her renal impairment?

B How would you confirm your diagnosis?

C How would you treat this condition?

A Interstitial nephritis secondary to chronic non-steroidal analgesic ingestion for back pain.

B Renal biopsy shows tubular necrosis with an eosinophilic infiltrate.

C Treatment is to stop the causative drug, start high dose oral steroids and treat the acute renal failure.

Acute interstitial nephritis classically presents with oliguric renal failure, fever, peripheral eosinophilia and eosinophiluria, and may include arthralgia. Drugs, especially non-steroidals are the commonest cause. Other drugs that may cause this condition include diuretics, heavy metals, e.g. gold and anticonvulsants.

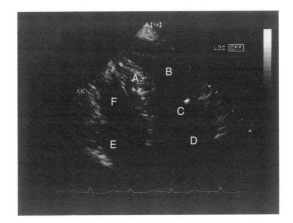

A Label structures A to F in the 2-D echocardiograph shown above.

B What abnormality is shown?

C What is the most likely underlying condition?

A

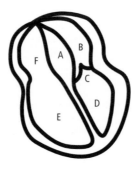

```
A = Interventricular septum
B = Left ventricular cavity
C = Mitral valve
D = Left atrial cavity
E = Right atrial cavity
F = Right ventricular cavity
```

B Asymmetrical septal hypertrophy (ASH).

C Hypertrophic obstructive cardiomyopathy.

The classical echocardiographic features of hypertrophic cardiomyopathy are asymmetrical septal hypertrophy (interventricular septum: posterior left ventricular wall ratio greater than 1.3:1) and systolic anterior motion of the mitral valve (SAM). The hypertrophy may be localized to anywhere within the left ventricle or may be generalized. There is a reduction in left ventricular cavity size and systolic obliteration of the cavity may occur.

A 22-year-old asthmatic female was brought into casualty short of breath. She gave a four-day history of fever and cough productive of green sputum. Her general practitioner had started her on oral antibiotics. On examination, she was tachypnoeic and had a widespread expiratory wheeze without evidence of focal consolidation.

Investigations gave the following results:

Sodium 135 mmol/l, potassium 4.6 mmol/l, urea 3.4 mmol/l, creatinine 120 µmol/l.

Hb 12.5 g/dl, WCC 14.6×10^9/l, Plts 240×10^9/l.

Arterial blood gases on air: pO_2 9.8 kPa, pCO_2 4.2 kPa, oxygen saturation 93%.

Chest radiograph showed hyperexpansion with flattened diaphragms.

Ward nurses called the house physician two hours later, as her oxygen saturation has dropped to 80%.

A Give the three likeliest causes of her deterioration.

B What immediate tests would you request?

A Exhaustion.
Segmental lung collapse due to mucous plugging.
Pneumothorax.

B Repeat arterial blood gases.
Chest radiograph would show up segmental collapse and pneumothorax.

Although a pneumothorax needs to be excluded, exhaustion is a more likely cause of the fall in oxygen saturation. A rising pCO_2 would change the management as the patient may then require assisted ventilation.

A 24-year-old male returned from a holiday to India with a two-week history of malaise, nausea, vomiting and rigors. He had a past medical history of jaundice three years previously following a trip to Africa. Clinically he had low-grade pyrexia and was icteric.

The following investigative results were recorded:

Hb 12.7 g/dl, WCC 8.5×10^9/l, Plts 180×10^9/l.

Sodium 132 mmol/l, potassium 4.8 mmol/l, urea 5.5 mmol/l, creatinine 120 μmol/l, AST 550 U/l, ALT 660 U/l, albumin 35 g/l, alkaline phosphatase 200 U/l.

HBsAg +, HBeAg −, Anti-HBe +.

A What further tests would you request to elucidate the cause of his jaundice?

B He has recently acquired a new sexual partner. Is he a high or low risk candidate for transmitting hepatitis B?

A IgM anti-HAV (hepatitis A).

Delta agent antibody.

Anti-HCV (hepatitis C virus detected by PCR).

His hepatitis B serology suggests chronic carrier status. He probably acquired hepatitis B after his previous trip to Africa. His current deterioration suggests acquisition of a new hepatitis virus such as delta agent infection associated with his hepatitis B infection. This is usually acquired by intravenous drug abuse. Hepatitis E infection is spread faeco-orally and is especially prevalent in the Indian subcontinent.

B He is at low risk of transmitting hepatitis B as antibodies to the e antigen of hepatitis B denotes decreased infectivity risk.

An 87-year-old female was admitted with a five-day history of increasing shortness of breath. She had a past medical history of long-standing hypertension. On examination she had a blood pressure of 190/100 mmHg. She had bibasal crepitations on auscultation and was started on a diuretic. The following day she spiked a temperature and complained of dysuria. Urine dipstick revealed the presence of blood and protein. She was commenced on empirical treatment for a presumed urinary tract infection.

Four days later the house physician is alarmed by the patient's latest electrolyte results:

On admission: sodium 145 mmol/l, potassium 4.0 mmol/l, urea 25 mmol/l, creatinine 424 µmol/l, bicarbonate 23 mmol/l.

Day 4: Sodium 143 mmol/l, potassium 3.9 mmol/l, urea 28 mmol/l, creatinine 630 µmol/l, bicarbonate 24 mmol/l.

A   Can you account for the change in her electrolyte results?

B   Give three other causes for this anomaly.

A Trimethoprim treatment for her urinary tract infection has caused a disproportionate rise in creatinine.

B Other causes of a disproportionately high creatinine: urea ratio include:
- Other drugs, e.g. cimetidine.
- Secondary to rhabdomyolysis.
- Low urea caused by liver disease, dialysis, pregnancy.
- Racial predisposition to a high creatinine, e.g. in Afro-Caribbean people.

Urinary creatinine is the sum of filtered and secreted creatinine. In normal individuals, the glomerular filtration rate accounts for over 90% of excreted creatinine. In patients with a serum creatinine over 400 µmol/l, however, secreted creatinine from the distal tubule accounts for a significant proportion of the excreted creatinine. Trimethoprim and cimetidine compete for this secretion: thus plasma creatinine rises but there is effectively no alteration in the glomerular filtration rate as measured by insulin clearance. Therefore, no specific treatment is necessary in the present case and the trimethoprim therapy may be continued, if it is deemed to be beneficial.

An active 60-year-old female had a history of rheumatic heart disease. She had remained largely asymptomatic until recently when she had noticed increasing exertional dyspnoea and presyncope. At cardiac catheterization she was found to have a left ventricular pressure of 240/15 mmHg in the presence of well preserved left ventricular function. The aortic pressure was 160/70 mmHg. There was no significant coronary artery disease. Transthoracic echocardiography had shown a peak pressure gradient of 110 mmHg.

A What is the diagnosis from the available data?

B What is the aortic valve gradient derived from cardiac catheterization?

C Why is there a discrepancy between the aortic valve pressure gradients derived by cardiac catheterization and echocardiography?

D What other valve parameter may be used to assess the severity of this condition?

A Severe rheumatic aortic stenosis.

B 80 mmHg (left ventricular (systole)-aortic pressure (systole)).

C The discrepancy between the aortic valve gradients obtained at echocardiography and at cardiac catheterization are a reflection of the different methods used in measurement. The gradient obtained at echocardiography is an instantaneous gradient, obtained by a measurement of the peak flow velocity across the aortic valve (using the Doppler principal). This is used in conjunction with the modified Bernoulli equation to derive the required gradient (Pressure difference, mmHg = 4 × [peak flow velocity, m/s]^2). The catheter gradient is a peak-to-peak pressure gradient, i.e. measuring the difference between the peak pressure in the left ventricle and that in the aorta (derived later following withdrawal of the catheter from the left ventricle into the aorta).

D Aortic valve area. Use of the continuity equation allows calculation of the valve area: orifice area (cm^2) = π × radius of left ventricular outflow tract^2 (cm^2) × subaortic peak velocity (m/s)/aortic peak velocity (m/s).

	Degree of aortic stenosis		
	Mild	Moderate	Severe
Peak flow velocity (m/s)	<3	3–4	>4
Peak instantaneous gradient (mmHg)	Negligible	35–65	>65
Valve area (cm^2)	>1.0	0.6–1.0	<0.6

A 25-year-old female was seen in clinic with a history of increasing shortness of breath on exertion. She had mild asthma as a child for which she used an inhaler. There was no other salient history although systemic enquiry revealed occasional bleeding per rectum since her first pregnancy.

The following lung function tests were obtained:

FEV$_1$ 2.00 l (predicted 2.13).

FVC 2.50 l (predicted 2.55).

TLC-He 4.75 l (predicted 4.84).

RV-He 1.55 l (predicted 1.95).

T$_L$CO 6.33 ml/min/mmHg (predicted 21.7).

KCO 1.75 min^{-1} (predicted 3.15).

What is the likeliest explanation for these lung function results?

Anaemia.

The reduction of the KCO together with a history of shortness of breath and rectal bleeding, suggests anaemia may be the underlying cause of this lady's breathing problems.

T_LCO (transfer factor) or D_LCO (diffusing factor) gives a measure of efficacy of gas transfer from alveoli to blood as measured by carbon monoxide. This measurement is thus dependent on the number of functioning alveoli and the state of their respective membranes, and the blood flow to the alveoli, a function of both the number of circulating red blood cells and the integrity of the alveolar capillary network. The KCO is an equivalent value to the T_LCO, but is corrected for lung volume (KCO = T_LCO/alveolar volume).

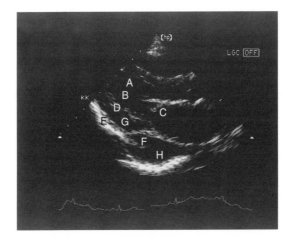

A 70-year-old male presented with a history of breathlessness, weight loss and haemoptysis. Clinical examination shows him to be clubbed. Chest examination reveals dullness to percussion at both lung bases with reduced breath sounds on auscultation. A transthoracic echocardiogram is performed and the 2-D parasternal long-axis view is shown.

Label the structures A to H in the 2-D echocardiograph shown above.

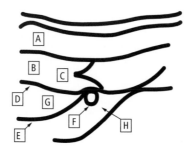

A.	Right ventricle
B.	Left ventricular cavity
C.	Mitral valve
D.	Left ventricular posterior wall
E.	Pericardium
F.	Descending aorta
G.	Pericardial effusion
H.	Pleural effusion

A pericardial effusion is seen in front of the echogenic pericardium and descending aorta and behind the left ventricular posterior wall. The pleural effusion is the echo-free space behind the left atrium and pericardium. Given the history, a malignant aetiology must be suspected, with a possible bronchial primary.

A 46-year-old male was seen in an outpatient clinic with a three-month history of weight loss and malaise. He had noted weakness of his legs, especially when climbing stairs or rising from a chair. In the previous two weeks he had developed a dry cough. He had stopped smoking 40 cigarettes a day over two years previously. On examination, he was found to be cachectic and appeared tanned. Neurologically he had evidence of proximal lower limb weakness.

The following investigative results were recorded:

Hb 10.5 g/dl, MCV 89 fl, WCC 5.5×10^9/l, Plts 170×10^9/l.

Sodium 140 mmol/l, potassium 2.4 mmol/l, urea 6.0 mmol/l, creatinine 100 μmol/l, bicarbonate 35 mmol/l, glucose 12 mmol/l.

Chest radiograph: unremarkable.

A What is the likely underlying diagnosis?

B What further tests would you request to support your diagnosis?

A Cushing's syndrome caused by ectopic ACTH production from an unknown primary tumour, either benign (e.g. carcinoid) or malignant (e.g. carcinoma of the bronchus).

B Serum ACTH and cortisol levels.
Challenge with corticotrophin releasing hormone (CRF).
High dose dexamethasone suppression test.
Bronchoscopy.
CT thorax and abdomen.

This man presents with weight loss, a proximal myopathy and excessive tanning, which together with a very low potassium and an alkalosis is highly suggestive of ectopic ACTH production, most probably from an oat cell bronchogenic carcinoma, despite the normal chest radiograph. Serum ACTH levels would be expected to be greater than 200 ng/l in the presence of a high cortisol level. Classically, ectopic ACTH tumours are not suppressed during high dose dexamethasone suppression, whereas the majority (90%) of pituitary-dependent steroid secreting tumours are suppressed to 50% of basal and most will show an exaggerated ACTH response to exogenous CRF.

A 28-year-old male was admitted with a reduced conscious level, photophobia and neck stiffness. He had declined rapidly over a day. On examination, he was drowsy but had a normal Glasgow Coma Scale score of 15. There was evidence of neck stiffness and he was Kernig's sign positive. The past medical history included a serious road traffic accident a year previously which had rendered him unconscious; he had suffered an episode of bacterial meningitis for three months following this.

The following investigative results were recorded:

Hb 13.6 g/dl, WCC 12.5×10^9/l, Plts 160×10^9/l.

Serum glucose 7 mmol/l.

CSF: 1000 leucocytes/mm^3 (mainly polymorphs), protein 3 g/l, glucose 2 mmol/l, Gram negative intracellular diplococci seen on microscopy.

He was commenced on high dose intravenous benzylpenicillin and made a good recovery. Prior to discharge he was noted to have a persistent nasal drip which on further questioning, he admitted to having had over the last eight months.

A What is the likely source of his nasal drip?

B What ward test could you use to confirm this?

A CSF rhinorrhoea from the previous skull fracture.

B CSF has a higher sugar content than normal nasal secretions and a simple dipstick test should highlight this.

A 35-year-old Indian female was admitted with sudden onset of weakness along her left-hand side. She had noticed her left leg dragging 12 hours earlier and eventually found she was unable to move her left arm. She also gave a two-month history of increasing fatigue, aching muscles and occasional night sweats. She had arrived from India three months earlier.

On examination, she was mildly pyrexial at 37.6°C. Blood pressure was 130/100 mmHg with sinus tachycardia. The cardiac apex was not displaced and was heaving in nature. There was a 4/6 ejection systolic murmur at the left sternal edge and over the aortic area radiating to both carotid arteries. Abdominal examination revealed a palpable spleen. Neurologically, she had a dense left-sided hemiparesis.

The following investigative results were recorded:

Hb 9.8 g/dl, MCV 85 fl, WCC 4.8×10^9/l, Plts 120×10^9/L, PT 15 s, APTT 31 s.

Sodium 135 mmol/l, potassium 4.8 mmol/l, urea 8.5 mmol/l, creatinine 150 μmol/l, albumin 38 g/l, ALT 55 IU/l, alkaline phosphatase 145 IU/l, total bilirubin 15 μmol/l.

CRP 10 mg/l, ESR 90 mm/h.

Echocardiogram: Mobile masses adherent to the aortic valve leaflets; peak instantaneous aortic valve gradient of 30 mmHg with trivial mitral regurgitation.

Blood cultures: no organism grown.

A What is the likely underlying diagnosis?

B What further tests would you perform?

A Systemic lupus erythematosus with Liebman–Sacks endocarditis.

B Serology for ANA, dsDNA, lupus anticoagulant, antiphospholipid (including anticardiolipin antibodies), TPHA/VDRL.
CT scan brain.

Sterile vegetations can accumulate on both the mitral and aortic valves in Liebman–Sacks endocarditis. These vegetations may embolize, as in this case, and lead to further complications, such as cerebral infarction. The vegetations can become infected; infective endocarditis is less likely in this case as the CRP is normal. The mild renal impairment and normochromic, normocytic anaemia are both consistent with SLE.

A 55-year-old male presented with a history of gradually increasing shortness of breath. He had first experienced problems three months earlier when he had begun to feel tired and listless. He had noticed difficulty in climbing stairs and in walking. He had developed difficulty in swallowing meat and had been restricted to a largely vegetarian diet. A week before presentation, he had a bout of haemoptysis. He was a life-long smoker, who had had tuberculosis as a young man.

On examination, he was cachectic. There were telangiectasiae present over his arms and chest, and red streaking over his metacarpophalyngeal (MCP) joints. Respiratory examination was unremarkable. Neurologically, he had proximal weakness in the upper and lower limbs. There was no change in reflexes or power after exercise.

The following investigative results were recorded:

Hb 10.1 g/dl, MCV 72 fl, W.C.C 9.5×10^9/l, Plts 160×10^9/l, ESR 70 mm/h.

Sodium 132 mmol/l, potassium 4.5 mmol/l, urea 2.2 mmol/l, creatinine 70 μmol/l, CK 850 IU/l, albumin 22 g/l, ALT 25 IU/l, bilirubin 10 μmol/l.

A What is the likely cause of his weakness?

B What further tests would you perform to confirm this?

A Dermatomyositis secondary to carcinoma of the bronchus.

B Nerve conduction studies/Electromyography (EMG).
Muscle biopsy.
Chest radiograph/bronchoscopy/CT thorax.

Dermatomyositis has the clinical features of polymyositis in addition to a characteristic rash, in this case manifested by telangiectasiae and streaking of the MCP joints. More characteristically, there may be a purple heliotrope rash present over the eyelids. There is an association with underlying malignancy, usually carcinoma of the bronchus or ovary. There is muscle weakness and tenderness of the proximal limb girdle and dysphagia occurs in 50%. The diagnosis is based on a high CPK/aldolase level together with a characteristic EMG pattern, which may show short polyphasic motor potentials, spontaneous fibrillation and high frequency repetitive discharges. Muscle biopsy may show necrosis, fragmentation and vacuolation of muscle fibres as well as the presence of B lymphocytes.

A 25-year-old female presented with a history of loose offensive stools and abdominal discomfort. In addition, she had noted an increasing tendency to painful muscle spasms.

Her initial investigations were as follows:

Hb 12.9 g/dl, WCC 6×10^9/l, Plts 529×10^9/l, MCV 62 fl, Haematocrit 0.4, MCH 19.8 pg, MCHC 32 g/dl. Blood film: target cells, Howell–Jolly bodies.

A What is the diagnosis?

B What further investigations are necessary?

C What is the cause of the Howell–Jolly bodies?

A Coeliac disease.

B Liver function tests, serum calcium and haematinic levels, duodenal biopsy.

C Howell–Jolly bodies are nuclear remnants. The spleen is responsible for removing these and their presence therefore indicates hyposplenism. The reason why this should occur in coeliac disease is currently unclear. Other causes of acquired hyposplenism include sickle cell anaemia, dermatitis herpetiformis (which may also occur in association with coeliac disease), essential thrombocythaemia, inflammatory bowel disease and Fanconi's anaemia.

This patient has symptoms that are classical for coeliac disease. Her muscle spasms may relate to hypocalcaemia consequent to the malabsorption. Many patients may, however, present incidentally with iron deficiency anaemia, macrocytosis or a blood film suggestive of hyposplenism without such symptoms. This lady has evidence of microcytic, hypochromic red cells suggestive of iron deficiency, in addition to Howell–Jolly bodies, indicating hyposplenism, both of which would be consistent with coeliac disease. Diagnosis requires the demonstration, on at least two small intestinal biopsies, of total villous atrophy, which reverses following a gluten-free diet.

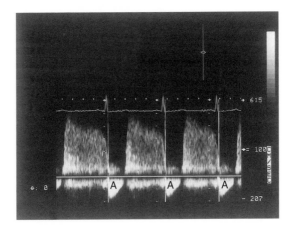

A 38-year-old male, over 180 cm tall, presented with shortness of breath on exertion and orthopnoea. On examination, he had a collapsing pulse and an early diastolic murmur audible at the left sternal edge in deep expiration. The first heart sound was normal in intensity. A continuous wave Doppler recording taken across the aortic valve at transthoracic echocardiography is shown above.

A What abnormal process is indicated by A in the above figure?

B What would be the underlying mechanism causing a mid-diastolic murmur in this context?

C What is the eponymous name given to a mid-diastolic murmur in this context?

A Abnormal flow in diastole directed towards the transducer (positioned at the apex). This would be consistent with aortic regurgitation.

B In significant aortic regurgitant, the regurgitant jet may cause the anterior mitral valve leaflet to oscillate between itself and the blood flow through the mitral valve during diastole. This fluttering of the anterior mitral valve leaflet in diastole with decreased diastolic excursion of the mitral valve leaflet may be recognized echocardiographically. Auscultation reveals a mid-diastolic murmur in addition to the early diastolic murmur of aortic regurgitation.

C The mid-diastolic murmur is known as the Austin–Flint murmur.

A 40-year-old female with long-standing rheumatoid arthritis was seen with a history of pyrexia, malaise, and a cough productive of green sputum. She had had frequent chest infections over the preceding few months. Her rheumatoid arthritis medications had recently been changed by her consultant but she couldn't remember her current therapy.

On examination, she was pyrexial at 37.5°C. Rubbery cervical and axillary lymph nodes were present. Respiratory examination revealed bronchial breathing at the left base. Abdominal examination revealed hepatosplenomegaly.

The following investigative results were recorded:

Hb 8.5 g/dl, WCC 2.5×10^9/l, Plts 60×10^9/l.

Sodium 135 mmol/l, potassium 4.5 mmol/l, urea 2.2 mmol/l, creatinine 90 µmol/l.

A Give a differential diagnosis for her haematological indices.

B Give four possible causes of the splenomegaly in this context.

A Felty's syndrome: seropositive rheumatoid arthritis with splenomegaly and neutropenia.
Lymphadenopathy, hepatomegaly, vasculitis, anaemia and thrombocytopenia may also occur in Felty's syndrome.
Pancytopenia secondary to azathioprine/cyclophosphamide.

B Rheumatoid arthritis.
Sjögren's disease secondary to rheumatoid arthritis.
Felty's syndrome.
Secondary amyloidosis.

A 25-year-old male had come for genetic counselling. He had recently married and was known to have vitamin D resistant (hypophosphataemic) rickets.

A What proportion of his sons may be affected?

B Which of his parents would have been affected?

A None, all his daughters will be affected however.

B Mother.

Vitamin D resistant rickets is an X-linked dominant condition. The table below illustrates the progeny of an affected male/normal female pairing, with the vitamin D resistance gene denoted by superscript 'r':

	X^r	Y
X	X^rX	XY
X	X^rX	XY

Sons may only acquire the gene from affected mothers:

	X	Y
X^r	X^rX	X^rY
X	XX	XY

A 21-year-old student presented with a one-week history of an inflamed right wrist joint, pyrexia and malaise. She had been diagnosed as having systemic lupus erythematosus three years earlier and was on steroid treatment. She had recently acquired a new sexual partner.

On examination, she was pyrexial at 38°C and had pustular, haemorrhagic lesions over her arms and legs. Her right wrist joint was hot, swollen and felt 'boggy'. A spleen tip was palpable on abdominal examination.

The following investigative results were recorded:

Hb 11.6 g/dl, MCV 88 fl, WCC 14.5×10^9/l, Plts 90×10^9/l, PT 15 s, APTT 44 s, ESR 90 mm/h, CRP 200 mg/l C3/C4: elevated.

Sodium 132 mmol/l, potassium 4.6 mmol/l, urea 8.4 mmol/l, creatinine 148 µmol/l, albumin 38 g/l, ALT 44 IU/l, alkaline phosphatase 90 IU/l.

A Give the likeliest cause of her deterioration.

B What further investigations would you perform to confirm this?

C What is the cause of her prolonged APTT?

D How would treat this patient?

A Gonococcal arthritis.

B Blood cultures.
Joint aspiration with Gram stain of synovial fluid and culture.
Culture of secretions from urethra, endocervix, rectum/pharynx, skin lesions.

C Lupus anticoagulant.

D High-dose intravenous benzylpenicillin.
Increase steroids as low platelet count suggests active lupus.
Contact tracing for gonorrhoea.

Symptomatic gonorrhoea is most often found in young females or homosexual males. The arthralgia is often asymmetrical and usually involves the upper limb. The pustular, haemorrhagic lesions are usually found on the limbs and the condition may be complicated by hepatitis or perihepatitis (Fitz–Hugh–Curtis syndrome), myocarditis and endocarditis. The deterioration is unlikely to be due to lupus alone in view of the characteristic rash in the context of a new sexual partner, and in view of the elevated CRP and complement titres.

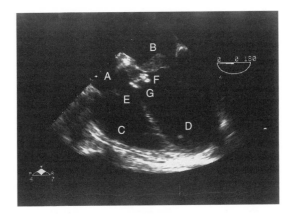

This 42-year-old male presented with a history lethargy and profuse nocturnal sweating. He had suffered an episode of transient visual loss in his right eye, which he described as a 'shutter being lowered across his eye'. On examination he was febrile. There was an early diastolic murmur audible at the left sternal edge with a pansystolic murmur audible at the apex and radiating to the axilla.

A What investigation is this?

B What are the structures marked A–F?

C What abnormalities are shown?

D What is the diagnosis?

A Transoesophageal echocardiography: it is conventional in this investigation to show the atria at the top of the picture with the ventricles at the bottom. The angle sector shown at the right of the frame shows this is a multiplane TOE probe in use.

B

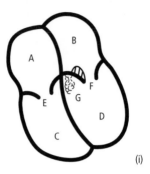

(i)

A Right atrium
B Left atrium
C Right ventricle
D Left ventricle
E Tricuspid valve
F Mitral valve

G Left ventricular outflow tract

C A large vegetation is seen attached to the anterior mitral valve leaflet. The posterior mitral valve leaflet is thickened and may also be involved. There are abnormal echos in the left ventricular outflow tract, which may suggest calcified vegetations in association with the aortic valve/aorto-mitral continuity.

D Infective endocarditis.

A 68-year-old male was re-referred to a cardiology outpatient clinic by his general practitioner with increasing shortness of breath on exertion and intermittent chest pains. He was last seen 10 years earlier for palpitations and mild angina, and was on diltiazem and procainamide. The chest pain was stabbing in nature and was worse on inspiration. On examination, he had a pansystolic murmur at the left sternal edge radiating to the axilla and on respiratory examination breath sounds were reduced at both bases with a stony dull percussion note at the right base.

The following results were noted:

Sodium 134 mmol/l, potassium 4.5 mmol/l, urea 5.6 mmol/l, creatinine 112 μmol/l.

Hb 10.5 g/dl, MCV 87 fl, WCC 6.5×10^9/l, Plts 160×10^9/l, ESR 80 mm/h, CRP 8 mg/l.

C3/C4: normal level.

Chest radiograph: bilateral elevated diaphragms with small lung volumes; right pleural effusion.

A What is the cause of his respiratory symptoms?

B What is the likely underlying cause of his condition?

C What further tests would you carry out to confirm your suspicions?

A Drug-induced lupus with restrictive lung defect.

B Long-term procainamide treatment.

C Serology for ANA, dsDNA, antihistone antibody.
Lung function tests.
CT scan thorax.
Bronchoscopy with transbronchial biopsy.

Drug-induced lupus is characterized by a homogenous ANA distribution. Unlike systemic lupus erythematosus, dsDNA is usually negative and complement titres are within normal limits. It is especially common with hydralazine and procainamide treatment but can occur with other drugs, e.g. chlorpromazine, isoniazid, phenytoin and the oral contraceptive pill. Respiratory involvement results in a restrictive lung picture on lung function testing; this is usually due to a primary diaphragmatic problem, leading to elevated diaphragms and reduced lung volumes, rather than lung fibrosis.

A 35-year-old male garage mechanic presented with haemoptysis. He had endured several bouts over the previous three months but was too scared to consult his general practitioner. He had recently noticed swelling of his ankles and was a heavy smoker.

On examination, he had a soft ejection systolic murmur audible at the left sternal edge with no radiation to the carotids arteries; the breath sounds were decreased at the right base with bronchial breathing.

The following results were noted:

Hb 11.6 g/dl, MCV 83 fl, WCC 7.5×10^9/l, Plts 450×10^9/l, ESR 80 mm/h.
Sodium 134 mmol/l, potassium 5.0 mmol/l, urea 12 mmol/l, creatinine 250 μmol/l.
Urine dipstick: protein + + blood + +.

A What is the differential diagnosis of the underlying condition?

B What further tests would you perform to elucidate the diagnosis?

A The differential diagnosis of a pulmonary-renal condition presenting with haemoptysis is wide: Goodpasture's syndrome/ SLE/ Wegener's granulomatosis/ Polyarteritis nodosa/ Essential cryoglobulinaemia/ Henoch–Schonlein purpura/ Right-sided subacute bacterial endocarditis with secondary glomerulonephritis and haemoptysis (due to recurrent septic pulmonary emboli).

B ANA/dsDNA/C3 & C4/
ANCA, antiglomerular basement membrane antibody
Cryoglobulin screen
CRP
Blood cultures
Echocardiography
Renal biopsy.

A 68-year-old female with dyspnoea and swollen ankles presented to the medical team on call. On examination, she was in controlled atrial fibrillation, with an audible pansystolic murmur at the left sternal edge with radiation to the axilla. A mid-diastolic murmur was audible at the apex, in the left lateral position.

At cardiac catheterization, the following data are obtained:

Pressure measurements (mmHg): Right atrial mean pressure 11; Right ventricular pressure 43/11; Left ventricular pressure: 139/8; Aortic pressure 140/80; Mitral valve gradient 8–11.

Left ventriculogram: good systolic function, mild mitral regurgitation

Coronary angiography: normal.

A What is the diagnosis?

B What further investigation is necessary?

A Severe mitral stenosis.

B Transoesophageal echocardiography: a detailed assessment of mitral valve morphology is necessary in order to assess suitability for mitral balloon valvuloplasty. This will depend on the degree of calcification of the mitral valve leaflets and subvalvar apparatus in addition to the degree of mitral regurgitation. Suboptimal results may be obtained in heavily calcified valves and there is the potential for any pre-existing mitral regurgitation to worsen following balloon valvuloplasty.

The severity of mitral stenosis can be assessed by transthoracic echocardiography and at cardiac catheterization. Cardiac catheterization allows estimation of the transmitral gradient (end-diastolic and mean) whilst echocardiography allows estimation of the mean transmitral gradient and mitral valve area. An end-diastolic mitral gradient of over 5 mmHg (or a mitral valve area less than 1 cm^2) denotes severe mitral stenosis.

A 68-year-old male attended a clinic for review of his hypertension and angina. He was taking diltiazem, frusemide and another pill for blood pressure, the name of which he could not recall. His blood pressure in clinic was 160/100 mmHg.

The following results were noted:

Hb 9.6 g/dl, MCV 104 fl, WCC 6.5 × 10⁹/l, Plts 220 × 10⁹/l.

Sodium 135 mmol/l, potassium 3.8 mmol/l, urea 6.5 mmol/l, creatinine 128 µmol/l, albumin 35 g/l, ALT 25 IU/l, total bilirubin 34 µmol/l, alkaline phosphatase 100 IU/l.

Blood film: reticulocytosis and spherocytes.

A What is the likely precipitant of this man's anaemia?

B How would you confirm your suspicions?

A He is likely to be taking α-methyldopa for his blood pressure.

B Coomb's test.
Serum haptoglobins.
Urine for haemosiderinuria.

α-methyldopa, along with mefanamic acid and ʟ-dopa, can induce the formation of autoantibodies against red cell membrane antigens. This causes a Coomb's positive haemolysis. If the haemolysis is severe enough, serum haptoglobins may fall and haemosiderinuria may be detectable.

A 33-year-old female with long-standing myaesthenia gravis was admitted with left loin pain, rigors and malaise. She was started on appropriate treatment for a presumed pyelonephritis. Two days later, the house physician was called to the ward as her breathing had markedly deteriorated.

He performed the following investigations:

Hb 13.6 g/dl, WCC 14.5×10^9/l, Plts 140×10^9/l.

Sodium 132 mmol/l, potassium 4.3 mmol/l, urea 2.5 mmol/l, creatinine 95 µmol/l.

Chest radiograph: unremarkable.

Oxygen saturation on air: 83%.

Give two causes for her deteriorating respiratory function.

Sepsis.
Aminoglycoside therapy for treatment of her presumed urinary tract infection has worsened her myaesthenia gravis.

Other factors that can exacerbate myaesthenic features include pregnancy, thyrotoxicosis, hypokalaemia and other drugs, e.g. propanolol, lignocaine and D-penicillamine.

A 50-year-old female was referred to a medical outpatient clinic with a history of a flu-like illness followed by vomiting and jaundice. She had noticed darkening of her urine. She had undergone a blood transfusion many years previously and had not been commenced on any new drugs recently. She did not drink any alcohol. On examination there were no signs of chronic liver disease. She had tender hepatomegaly.

Her initial investigations were as follows:

Hb 14 g/dl, WCC 4×10^9/l, Plts 104×10^9/l, MCV 92 fl.

Bilirubin 200 μmol/l, alkaline phosphatase 170 IU/l, AST 1050 IU/l, ALT 700 IU/l, total protein 63 g/l, albumin 31 g/l, globulins 33 g/l, gamma GT 200 IU/l.

Hepatitis (A, B and C): EBV and CMV serology negative.

Autoantibody screen: ANF positive (1 in 160).

Abdominal ultrasound: normal

Liver biopsy: heavy mononuclear chronic inflammatory infiltrate in the portal tracts with piece-meal necrosis; hepatocytes show balloon degeneration; bridging fibrosis is present with nodular regeneration and micronodular cirrhosis.

A What is the diagnosis?

B How would you manage this patient?

A Autoimmune (lupoid) chronic active hepatitis.

B Prednisolone, orally with the subsequent use of azathioprine. The response to therapy can be followed by repeat liver function tests initially and then a further liver biopsy.

This diagnosis is suggested by the elevated liver transaminases, positive antinuclear factor (ANF) and liver histology. The latter is characterized by a mononuclear inflammatory infiltrate in the portal and periportal areas of the liver with the subsequent development of piece-meal necrosis, bridging fibrosis and liver cirrhosis. The presence of smooth muscle antibodies may also be a useful diagnostic feature.

A 40-year-old male was referred to the medical clinic having had a systolic murmur noted by his general practitioner. He had noted an increased tendency to exertional dyspnoea over the previous year and recently had a presyncopal episode whilst running for a bus. On clinical examination, he was found to have an ejection systolic murmur audible at the left sternal edge and the left ventricular apex. No clicks were audible. At left heart catheterization, the following pressure recordings were taken:

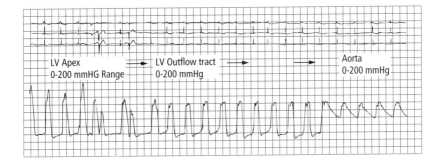

A What is your interpretation of the pressure recordings presented?

B What is the diagnosis?

C What characteristic features would you expect to see on transthoracic echocardiography?

A A pressure gradient is apparent between the left ventricular apex and left ventricular outflow tract.

B Hypertrophic obstructive cardiomyopathy.

C The most striking echocardiographic features of this condition include asymmetrical septal hypertrophy (with interventricular septum: posterior left ventricular wall ratio greater than 1.3:1) and systolic anterior motion of the mitral valve.

Hypertrophic cardiomyopathy is an hereditary condition which may result in an abnormal thickening of the myocardium of the left and/or right ventricle, classically resulting in asymmetrical septal hypertrophy (60% cases), although concentric (30%) or distal (10%) hypertrophy may also occur. It may present with chest pain, shortness of breath on exertion, syncope and sudden death. Hypertrophic cardiomyopathy is the commonest cause of sudden death in adolescence. A left ventricular outflow tract gradient occurs in 25% of cases although presence *per se* does not indicate a greater risk of sudden death. The risk factors for this include a family history for sudden death, recurrent syncope, frequent non-sustained ventricular tachycardia, exercise hypotension and specific genotypes.

A 28-year-old male was admitted to the intensive care unit with a haemorrhagic rash and sepsis. His blood pressure remained unresponsive to fluid and inotropic resuscitation.

The following investigations are available:

Hb 10.5 g/dl, WCC 14×10^9/l, Plts 90×10^9/l.

Sodium 130 mmol/l, potassium 4.5 mmol/l, urea 1.2 mmol/l, creatinine 80 μmol/l.

Random cortisol 240 nmol/l.

A What is the cause of this man's continued hypotension?

B What is the mechanism for your answer to **A**?

C What further confirmatory tests would you carry out?

D What additional treatment may restore his haemodynamic stability?

A Acute adrenal insufficiency.

B Meningococcal sepsis causing adrenal infarction (Waterhouse–Friedrichsen syndrome).

C Short tetracosactrin test.

D Intravenous hydrocortisone.

A random cortisol of less than 280 nmol/l is suggestive of adrenal insufficiency, but further confirmation is provided by the short tetracosactrin test. A normal test should show a cortisol of >580 nmol/l with a rise of >170 nmol/l, 30 min after a 250-µg IM injection of tetracosactrin. Further confirmation of infarction of the adrenals may be sought by CT/MRI scan of the abdomen.

Intravenous hydrocortisone by infusion of 4 mg per hour (or 100 mg over 24 hours) or intramuscular hydrocortisone 100 mg every six hours provides an average stable plasma cortisol of 100 nmol/l, which is usual for septic or perioperative patients. Intravenous hydrocortisone boluses are NOT appropriate in adrenal insufficiency, as cortisol levels fall to low levels after only a few minutes. The use of intravenous boluses may be appropriate in other conditions (e.g. asthma) where patients have a normal pituitary adrenal axis. Treatment with high dose hydrocortisone as above provides both mineralocorticoid and glucocorticoid effects.

A 49-year-old male presented with intermittent symptoms of dizziness, lack of energy and incoherency in speech over a period of four months. He had been commenced on a β-adrenoceptor blocker for hypertension six months previously. An ECG showed the presence of a sinus bradycardia. A 24-h tape was organized and a representative set of ECG recordings from this are shown below:

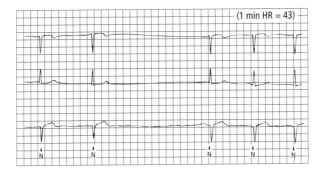

(1 min HR = 43)

A Comment on the ECG recording illustrated.

B What would your management of this patient be?

A Sinus bradycardia with sinus arrest producing sinus pauses of over 3 s (sinus node disease).

B Stop the β-adrenoceptor blocker and repeat the 24-h tape. Exclude hypothyroidism. If the pauses remain and the patient remains symptomatic, a permanent pacemaker will be required.

An 87-year-old female underwent a routine preoperative assessment by the surgical house physician for a total hip replacement. He noticed that she was pale and had a gravelly voice. She was in slow atrial fibrillation and was taking long-term digoxin therapy. She had bilateral pleural effusions and ascites.

He performed the following investigations:

Hb 10.5 g/dl, MCV 102 fl, WCC 7.5×10^9/l, Plts 170×10^9/l.

Sodium 120 mmol/l, potassium 4.0 mmol/l, urea 1.2 mmol/l, creatinine 95 μmol/l.

A What is the likely cause of her macrocytic anaemia?

B What is the mechanism of her hyponatraemia?

A Hypothyroidism.

B Syndrome of inappropriate antidiuretic hormone secretion (SIADH).

Some of the commonly presenting features of hypothyroidism are exemplified in the above case. The anaemia can be normocytic, microcytic (when it is usually associated with menorrhagia) or macrocytic (associated with vitamin B_{12} deficiency). Hypothyroidism is one of the predisposing causes of SIADH, as thyroxine is required for normal free water clearance by the kidney (as is cortisol).

The medical registrar was asked to review a patient on a psychiatric ward following a *grand mal* seizure witnessed by the nursing staff. The patient had been diagnosed as schizophrenic and had been started on antipsychotic medication five days earlier. He had been nonspecifically unwell for the last two days and had taken to remaining in his bed.

The patient was drowsy and not compliant in giving any further history. On examination, he was pyrexial at 38°C and had a sinus tachycardia. He was generally stiff but markedly so in the neck. Further examination, including full neurological assessment was unremarkable.

The following investigations were obtained:

Hb 11.7 g/dl, WCC 14.5 × 10^9/l, Plts 120 × 10^9/l.

Sodium 138 mmol/l, potassium 4.5 mmol/l, urea 4.8 mmol/l, creatinine 95 µmol/l, glucose 4.0 mmol/l, CPK 600 IU/l, albumin 32 g/l, ALT 25 IU/l, bilirubin 9 µmol/l, alkaline phosphatase 95 IU/l.

A What is the differential diagnosis of his condition?

B Give two causes of his raised CPK.

C What further tests would you perform to elucidate the diagnosis?

A Neuroleptic malignant syndrome.
  Meningitis.
  Encephalitis.
  Sub-arachnoid haemorrhage.
  Cerebral abscess.
  Catatonia.

B Neuroleptic malignant syndrome.
  Post *grand mal* seizure.

C CT scan brain followed by lumbar puncture with microscopy and culture of cerebrospinal fluid (CSF).

Neuroleptic malignant syndrome classically develops as an idiosyncratic reaction 1–3 days after starting phenothiazine or butyrophenone therapy. It is characterized by a change in conscious level, hyperpyrexia and muscular rigidity. The creatinine kinase is elevated due to muscle damage, and the myoglobin release that follows can lead to acute renal failure. Other sequelae include cardiac and respiratory failure. Treatment involves cooling down, rehydration and ventilatory support if required. Intravenous dantrolene and dopamine agonists, e.g. bromocriptine, have been shown to be of some benefit.

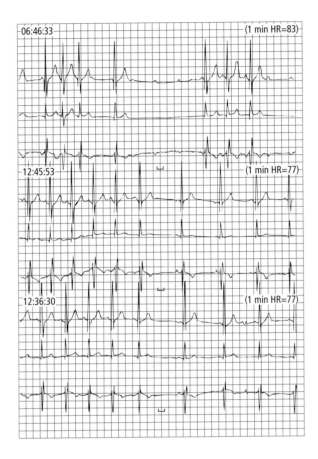

A 28-year-old male described an episode during which he became acutely dizzy. He was found by his wife lying on his bed shaking. He had not been incontinent. On examination, his pulse was 60/min and blood pressure was 120/80 mmHg. The initial investigations revealed a normal CT scan of the head and EEG. Representative examples of his 24-h tape are shown above.

A Comment on the ECG recordings illustrated.

B What would your management of this patient be?

A Diffuse conducting system disease with examples of sinus arrest with escape beats from a separate atrial focus (note different P wave axis); Mobitz type II second degree atrioventricular block leading to complete heart block (ventricular standstill).

B A permanent pacemaker is indicated.

A 52-year-old male was seen in an outpatient clinic with headaches, which were worst in the morning. On further questioning, he gave a three-month history of fatigue, feeling excessively cold, and of decreased libido. A month prior to being seen, he had begun to experience trouble in sleeping, mainly because of increasing nocturia.

The following investigations were carried out:

Sodium 150 mmol/l, potassium 4 mmol/l, urea 2 mmol/l, creatinine 68 μmol/l, glucose 5 mmol/l, urine osmolality: 102 mOsmol/l.

A What is this patient's calculated plasma osmolality?

B Comment on the result.

C In view of the above history, what is the likely cause of this man's problems?

D What treatment is required?

A Plasma osmolality
$$= (2 \times [Na]) + (2 \times [K]) + Urea + Glucose$$
$$= 300 + 8 + 2 + 5$$
$$= 315 \, mOsmol/l \, (normal \, range \, 275-295).$$

B The calculated osmolality is raised consistent with diabetes insipidus.

C Pituitary or hypothalamic tumour.

This patient is producing excessively dilute urine in the presence of an increased plasma osmolality, suggesting a deficiency of, or a lack of activity of, antidiuretic hormone (ADH). The ensuing diabetes insipidus may be of a central nervous or nephrogenic origin. The nephrogenic variety may be caused by a variety of factors, including hypocalcaemia and hypokalaemia. Antidiuretic hormone (ADH) is produced in hypothalamic neurones, and is transported for storage in the posterior pituitary, via axons in the pituitary stalk. Central diabetes insipidus may be caused by a lack of hypothalamic production of ADH, due to, e.g., hypothalamic tumour/granuloma or a pituitary tumour causing compression of the pituitary stalk. The presentation with early morning headaches is typical of raised intracranial pressure, suggestive of a space-occupying lesion. Fatigue and the feeling of excessive coldness may be due to hypothyroidism secondary to lack of TSH, similarly the decreased libido would be secondary to reduction in FSH/LH secretion.

D DDAVP.

An elderly farmer was referred to an outpatient clinic with a history of falls. He denied any specific difficulties and was unable to give a detailed description of these episodes. There was a past medical history of ischaemic heart disease. The physical examination was unremarkable. His 12-lead ECG recording is shown below:

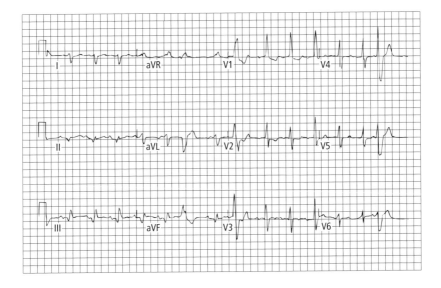

A Describe the abnormalities demonstrated on the ECG.

B What treatment is indicated?

A Right axis deviation and right bundle branch block (left posterior hemiblock); first degree heart block; ventricular ectopic beats; sinus rhythm; inferior Q waves (old inferior myocardial infarction); bifid P waves.

B Trifasicular block in the presence of a history of syncopal episodes is an indication for a permanent pacemaker.

An 82-year-old female was admitted with diarrhoea and dehydration. She gave an eight-month history of passing up to 10 stools/day. The stool was described as being offensive smelling and difficult to flush away. On examination, she was cachectic, and had proximal leg weakness with normal reflexes and sensation.

The following results are available:

Sodium 133 mmol/l, potassium 3.8 mmol/l, urea 4.0 mmol/l, creatinine 90 μmol/l, albumin 30 g/l, bilirubin 8 μmol/l, AST 10 IU/l, alkaline phosphatase 190 IU/l, calcium 1.8 mmol/l, phosphate 0.8 mmol/l.

Hb 8.7 g/dl, WCC 9×10^9/l, Plts 340×10^9/l, MCV 82 fl, PT 38 s, APTT 85 s.

A What is the likeliest cause of her clotting abnormality?

B How might you explain her leg weakness?

A Vitamin K deficiency.

B Osteomalacia secondary to vitamin D deficiency.

The history of offensive diarrhoea that is difficult to flush away would be compatible with steatorrhoea. The latter is accompanied by malabsorption of fat soluble vitamins A, D, E and K, manifested in this case by vitamin K deficient coagulopathy and osteomalacia (note the decreased calcium, the raised alkaline phosphatase and the proximal leg weakness).

The investigations below were from a patient with abnormal liver function tests (normal ranges are shown in parentheses):
Caeruloplasmin 0.04 g/l (0.2–0.6 g/l), total serum copper 5 μmol/l (11–22 μmol/l), 24 h urinary copper 1.2 mg/24 h (0.01–0.06 mg/24 h).

A What is the likeliest diagnosis in view of the above tests?

B Give a differential diagnosis.

C What definitive laboratory test would you carry out to confirm your answer to **A**?

A Wilson's disease.

B Primary biliary cirrhosis/ Very prolonged biliary obstruction/ Familial intrahepatic cholestasis.

C Urinary rise in copper excretion in response to penicillamine.
Delayed rate of radioactive copper incorporation into caeruloplasmin.

Decreased caeruloplasmin levels are found in a variety of diseases causing severe liver dysfunction. Increased urinary copper excretion is seen in primary biliary cirrhosis (PBC), prolonged biliary obstruction and familial intrahepatic cholestasis. The very low caeruloplasmin levels above, however, are highly suggestive of Wilson's disease.

The definitive laboratory test for Wilson's disease is the rate of incorporation of copper into caeruloplasmin, although this is rarely performed. The absence of Kayser–Fleischer rings is highly suggestive that the diagnosis is not Wilson's disease, although their presence is not pathognomonic of this disorder, as they are also found in other liver diseases, e.g. PBC. A liver biopsy is not diagnostic as the copper content/wet weight of liver is raised in all of the above disorders.

The following full blood count was carried out on a female inpatient with AIDS, who presented with HIV related nephropathy:

Hb 12.1 g/dl, Plts 33×10^9/l, MCV 88.8 fl, RCC 3.85×10^{12}/l, WCC 2.0×10^9/l, (neutrophils 1.6×10^9/l, lymphocytes 0.2×10^9/l), PT 14 s, APTT 33 s, TT 17 s, fibrinogen 2.1 g/l.

What is the likeliest cause of the low platelet count?

Autoimmune thrombocytopenia associated with HIV disease.

In view of the normal haemoglobin, bone marrow suppression due to lymphoma or drugs (e.g. AZT) is unlikely. Anti-platelet antibodies associated with HIV disease are widely reported.

A 35-year-old male was investigated for a three-month history of haemoptysis and left-sided pleuritic pain. The loss of blood was usually no more than a tablespoonful streaking the sputum but two days prior to being seen he had coughed up a large quantity of fresh blood. The pleuritic pain always accompanied a bout of haemoptysis and often persisted for up to a week.

A screen of tests was carried out including the following lung function tests:

FEV_1 2.90 l (predicted 3.2)
FVC 3.75 l (predicted 3.95)
TLC-He 6.95 l (predicted 7.05)
T_LCO 30.2 ml/min/mmHg (predicted 25.2)
KCO 7.4/min (predicted 5.3)

Explain the above lung function results.

Pulmonary haemorrhage.

The rise in T_LCO and KCO can be ascribed to the recent large haemoptysis, which was most probably the result of a pulmonary haemorrhage. This man's problems were due to a pulmonary arteriovenous malformation.

A 15-year-old Indian female was referred to the cardiology clinic with an audible systolic murmur that had been found incidentally by her general practitioner. She had noted pain in her legs recently during school physical education lessons.

At cardiac catheterization, the following pressure measurements (mmHg) were obtained:

Right atrium mean 2, right ventricle 28/4, pulmonary artery 27/12, left ventricle 120/4, ascending aorta 120/70, descending aorta 90/70.

A What is the diagnosis?

B What is the usual presentation in an adult?

C What features would you expect on her chest X-ray?

D Would you offer this patient advice concerning antibiotic prophylaxis prior to dental procedures?

A Coarctation of the aorta.

B Coarctation of the aorta may be entirely asymptomatic, usually being sought in adults with hypertension. Left untreated it may present as congestive cardiac failure, aortic rupture/dissection, endocarditis (on an associated bicuspid aortic valve)/endarteritis or cerebral haemorrhage (in association with berry aneurysms). It is also associated with Turner's syndrome.

C Cardiomegaly, dilatation of the ascending aorta, post-stenotic dilatation of the aorta (which in combination with a dilated left subclavian artery produces the reverse '3' sign), rib notching (which may be unilateral or bilateral, depending on the site of the coarctation in relation to the origin of the left subclavian artery).

D There is a theoretical risk of endocarditis presenting on an associated bicuspid aortic valve or endarteritis presenting at the site of the coarctation (although this is less common). Antibiotic prophylaxis should therefore be discussed with the patient.

A routine full blood count was carried out on a patient with AIDS in clinic. He was on rifabutin, ciprofloxacin, ranitidine and zidovudine treatment.
Hb 8.7 g/dl, MCV 116.6 fl, Plts 165×10^9/l, WCC 1.7×10^9/l: neutrophils 1.0×10^9/l, lymphocytes 0.4×10^9/l.

What is the likeliest cause of his macrocytosis?

Macrocytosis secondary to zidovudine therapy.

The medical registrar on duty was asked to review a 50-year-old female on the general surgical ward with a history of carcinoma of the stomach, which had been excised two weeks previously. She had become acutely dyspnoeic. A chest radiograph had shown bilateral pulmonary atelectasis. The ECG is shown below:

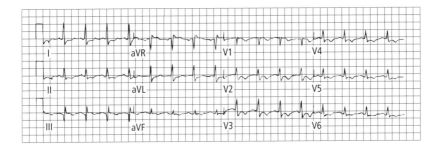

A Describe the ECG abnormalities demonstrated.

B What is the most likely diagnosis?

A Sinus tachycardia, right bundle branch block, $S_IQ_{III}T_{III}$ pattern (S wave in lead I, Q wave in lead III, T wave inversion in lead III), T wave inversion in the chest leads (right ventricular strain pattern) and inferior leads.

B Acute pulmonary embolism.

Although none of the ECG abnormalities listed above are entirely diagnostic of pulmonary embolism, their coexistence provides compelling evidence for the diagnosis. Atrial dysrrhythmias have also been described in pulmonary embolism.

A 50-year-old female was admitted to the orthopaedic ward following a fall.

The results of her initial investigations were as follows:.

Hb 11.3 g/dl, WCC 5.2 × 10^9/l, Plts 171 × 10^9/l, MCV 101 fl, MCH 39.9 pg, MCHC 35.3 g/dl, PT 30 s.
Blood film: target cells, burr cells, acanthocytes.

A What is the underlying cause of her blood test results?

B What confirmatory tests would you request?

A Alcoholic liver disease: gives rise to target cells, acanthocytes and round macrocytes and a coagulopathy.
Renal impairment: burr cells are a feature of renal failure.

B Liver function tests (including gamma GT), blood alcohol, urea and electrolytes.

A 28-year-old, HIV positive male presented in casualty with abdominal pain, decreased appetite, nausea and vomiting. He was on gancyclovir, cotrimoxazole, rifabutin, ethambutol, clarithromycin, salbutamol, cimetidine, methadone and didanosine (DDI), 200 mg b.d. Clinical examination and a plain abdominal radiograph were unremarkable.

The results of his blood tests are shown:

Sodium 141 mmol/l, potassium 4.6 mmol/l, urea 11.4 mmol/l, creatinine 153 µmol/l, alkaline phosphatase 468 IU/l, amylase 473 IU/l, calcium 2.1 mmol/l, phosphate 1.5 mmol/l.

A What is the cause of his abdominal pain?

B What has precipitated the above?

A Pancreatitis.

B DDI with cimetidine.

DDI is a nucleoside analogue used to delay progression of AIDS. DDI therapy is associated with discrete pathological changes within the pancreas, which may result in a hyperosmolar non-ketotic diabetic state or, as in this case, manifest as pancreatitis. This is likely with higher doses of DDI (200–750 mg/daily) and with the associated use of H_2 blockers, such as cimetidine, and proton pump inhibitors. The treatment of choice is stopping the DDI and treating the pancreatitis conservatively.

A 38-year-old female presented to her general practitioner with a six-month history of galactorrhoea and headaches. She last had a period two years earlier. Two months previously, the vision in her right eye had begun to deteriorate. Physical examination revealed a left upper quadrantinopia with fullness of the discs, the remainder of the examination being unremarkable.

The following results were recorded:

Hb 11.6 g/dl, WCC 6×10^9/l, Plts 280×10^9/l.

Sodium 132 mmol/l, potassium 4.3 mmol/l, urea 5.4 mmol/l, creatinine 105 μmol/l.

Thyroid function: TSH and T4 normal, cortisol normal.

Prolactin: 150 000 mU/l.

A What is the differential diagnosis?

B How would you confirm your diagnosis?

C How would you treat this patient?

A Macroprolactinoma.
Chromophobe adenoma with compression of pituitary stalk (this is unlikely in patients with a prolactin level in excess of 6000 mU/l).

B CT/MRI pituitary gland.

C Bromocriptine or cabergoline.
Surgical excision of tumour followed by postoperative radiotherapy if necessary.
Post-operative replacement of thyroxine and cortisol.

The history of amenorrhoea and galactorrhoea is suggestive of over-production of prolactin. This may occur either through a prolactin secreting tumour, or by compression of the pituitary stalk, preventing dopamine, made in the hypothalamic nuclei, from reaching the posterior pituitary and inhibiting prolactin production. The level of prolactin in the case presented above is highly suggestive of a prolactinoma, as stalk compression will rarely give prolactin levels > 3000 mU/l. The history of headaches and full discs is suggestive of raised intracranial pressure; this together with the left upper quadrantinopia is suggestive of an intracranial mass impinging on the right lower optic radiation. For a pituitary tumour to produce this visual loss, it would suggest suprasellar extension with invasion of the right middle cranial fossa.

Bromocriptine, a dopamine D_2 receptor agonist with weak antagonism at D_1 receptors, lowers prolactin levels, restores gonadal function, stops galactorrhoea and if a prolactinoma is present will cause it to shrink. Newer agents, such as cabergoline and quinagolide, also perform this function and have some advantages. Due to the lack of response to these drugs and the extent of invasion of this tumour, removal was performed surgically via a right frontal craniotomy, although smaller pituitary tumours may be removed via a transphenoidal approach.

A 65-year-old female was seen as a follow-up case in a cardiology outpatient clinic. She had a history of mitral valve replacement with a Starr–Edwards prosthesis 10 years previously. Her 12-lead ECG is shown below:

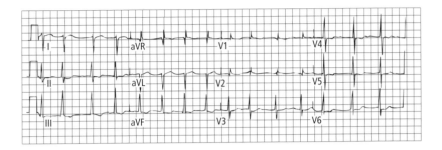

A What ECG abnormalities are present?

B What drugs would you anticipate this patient to be taking?

A Atrial fibrillation; right axis deviation with right bundle branch block pattern; 'reversed tick' appearance or ST segment sagging indicative of the digitalis effect.

B Digitalis and warfarin.

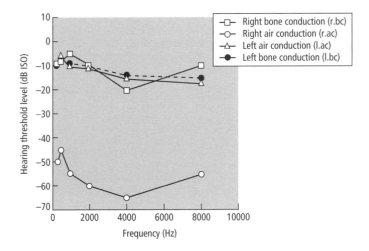

The audiogram presented above is taken from a 65-year-old male complaining of deafness progressing over the last month.

A What hearing defect is illustrated on the audiogram?

B Give a differential diagnosis.

A Unilateral conduction deafness affecting the right ear.

B Meatal obstruction, e.g. secondary to foreign body or carcinoma.
Middle ear effusion.
Ossicular discontinuity secondary to disease or injury.

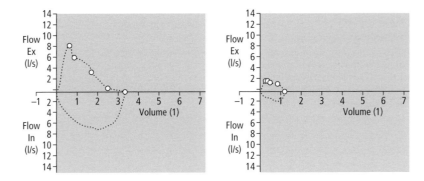

The flow–volume loop shown above right is that of a 29-year-old female, three months after a prolonged ITU admission. She required intubation and prolonged ventilation for the after effects of chicken-pox pneumonitis and subsequent septicaemia. For comparison, the flow–volume loop of a normal male, weighing 105 kg and 180 cm tall, is shown above left.

A What comments would you make about this patient's flow–volume loop?

B What underlying pathology may account for the above abnormality?

A The very small lung volume may suggest a small stature, in this case, height 155 cm and weight 44 kg. There is obvious severe restriction to inspiration and expiration suggestive of restrictive and obstructive disease.

B Acute adult respiratory distress syndrome, secondary to chicken-pox pneumonitis and sepsis, resulted in severe lung fibrosis in this particular patient, and hence the restrictive element of the flow–volume loop shown above. The obstructive pattern may have been due to tracheal stenosis as a result of long-term intubation.

A 36-year-old female was diagnosed as having Cushing's disease 18 months previously. She had been treated surgically by bilateral total adrenalectomy, the histology of the excised glands revealing hyperplasia of the adrenal cortex with some nodularity present. She was subsequently treated with cortisone acetate and 9α-fludrocortisone. She was re-referred to a medical outpatient clinic with pigmentation of the face, that had gradually increased over the preceding six months. She had noticed increasing tiredness. Her blood pressure was 150/70 mmHg. There were normal visual fields.

Her subsequent investigations are detailed below:

Plasma ACTH concentrations (ng/l):

Day	Time	ACTH
1	Midnight	470
2	09.00 hours	330
3	Midnight	640
4	09.00 hours	270

Chest and skull radiographs: normal

A What does the change in plasma ACTH values indicate?

B What is the diagnosis?

A Hypersecretion of ACTH.

B Nelson's syndrome.

The previous method for treating Cushing's disease was bilateral total adrenalectomy. In almost 10% of cases this resulted in the hypersecretion of ACTH with the subsequent development of Nelson's syndrome. This is because ACTH is cosecreted with MSH from pituitary adenomas which are no longer suppressed by adrenal steroids. Surgical removal of a pituitary microadenoma is now the first line of treatment.

Some suppression can be seen in this patient's ACTH level after his 06.00 hours dose of cortisone acetate.

A 50-year-old male had a long-standing history of coronary heart disease and refractory ventricular tachycardia. He had been treated with oral amiodarone and more recently had an automatic implantable cardioverter-defibrillator (AICD) inserted. He was admitted with a history of palpitations, with a blood pressure of 120/80 mmHg. A subsequent 12-lead ECG was taken which is shown below.

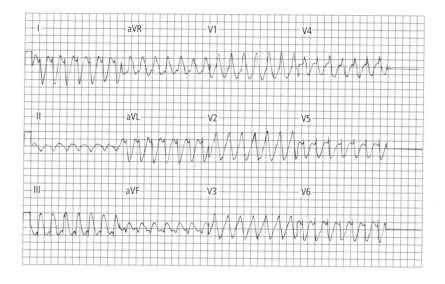

A What is the ECG diagnosis?

B What would you consider to be the most favourable method of treating this ECG abnormality?

A The ECG shows a regular broad complex tachycardia with atrioventricular dissociation and concordance of the QRS complexes. This appearance would be consistent with ventricular tachycardia.

B The ventricular rate is 168/min. The failure of the AICD to cardiovert may indicate unit dysfunction or that the ventricular rate at which the device is set to activate has not been exceeded. This can be assessed by interrogating the device; pace termination or cardioversion can then be activated externally.

A Extradural bleed
B Sub-dural bleed
C Sub-arachnoid bleed
D Cerebral venous sinus thrombosis
E Internal carotid artery dissection
F Vertebral artery dissection
G Wallenberg's syndrome
H Locked-in syndrome
I Inter-nuclear opthalmoplegia
J De-cerebrate posturing
K Coning

For each patient below choose the **SINGLE** most likely match from the above list of options. Each option may be used once, more than once or not at all.

1 A 30-year-old female presents with collapse and a reduced Glasgow Coma Scale (GCS). She had seen her GP two weeks previously with a history of new onset vertigo and had been prescribed a vestibular sedative. On the day of admission she complained of severe neck pain, increased vertigo, nausea and vomiting prior to her collapse.

2 A 56-year-old male presents to casualty with vertigo. Three days previously he had noticed sudden onset vertigo, transient diplopia, drooping of the left eyelid, severe nausea and vomiting. Examination revealed a left-sided ptosis, nystagmus in all directions of gaze and loss of pain over the right hand side of his body.

3 A 67-year-old male presents with collapse. The medical registrar was asked to see him on ITU. On examination he was intubated and ventilated. He had pinpoint pupils. Fundoscopy was normal. He was tetraparetic with extensor plantars. He was awake and alert but only able to blink and look up and down.

4 A 22-year-old male was on the rehabilitation unit after a road traffic accident. He had had neurosurgical decompression of a left fronto-temporal extradural bleed 4 days previously. On examination he had a dilated left pupil which did not respond to light. There were roving eye movements.

Corneal and doll's eye reflexes were intact. He was breathing via a tracheostomy. The upper limbs were extended and extended further to painful stimuli. The lower limbs were also extended with increased tone and extensor plantars.

5 A 21-year-old female presents with a three-month history of unsteadiness on walking and sensory disturbance over the right side of her face. A year previously, she had become bed-bound due to a gradual increase in stiffness and weakness in her legs. Examination on this occasion, showed a right afferent pupillary defect with visual acuity of 6/60 on the right and 6/6 on the left. On looking to the left she had nystagmus of the left eye and the right eye was unable to adduct fully. On looking to the right there was nystagmus of the right eye and the left eye was unable to adduct. There was further nystagmus on looking up or down.

6 The medical registrar was urgently bleeped to the ITU. A 28-year-old patient who was intubated and ventilated had developed new neurological signs. The ITU nurses had also noticed a steady rise in blood pressure and a new onset bradycardia.

7 A 33-year-old male presents to casualty. During intercourse an hour earlier he had noted a sudden headache over the back of this head. He had become nauseous and had vomited. He reported transient diplopia at the onset of the headache, which had resolved.

8 The medical registrar was asked to give an opinion on the obstetric ward. A 20-year-old female had given birth two days earlier to a daughter whilst stowed away as an illegal immigrant in a container lorry at Dover. The baby was doing well but the mother complained of a severe headache and had had a *grand mal* seizure that morning.

9 The medical registrar was asked to review the CT brain scan on a 23-year-old male who had fallen over whilst drunk. The patient had been found with a reduced GCS. There was an associated fracture of the right temporal area of the skull. There were no focal neurological signs.

1, F The sudden presentation with collapse is very suggestive of a vascular event. The combination of vertigo with nausea and vomiting is suggestive of a brain-stem localization. The severe neck pain is indicative of arterial dissection. The likeliest scenario is vertebral artery dissection causing a small brain stem stroke and thus the original history of vertigo. The acute presentation two weeks later is due to intraluminal clot formation at the site of the dissection causing a further stroke.

2, G This is a classical history of Wallenberg's (lateral medullary) syndrome due to posterior inferior cerebellar artery (PICA) occlusion. The symptoms and signs are due to involvement of the lateral medullary structures including the vestibular nuclei, dorsal motor nucleus of the vagal nerve, sympathetic tract and spinothalamic tract.

3, H Pin-point pupils are suggestive of either opiate analgesia or a mid-brain/pontine localization. The tetraparesis and extensor plantars suggest involvement of the corticospinal, corticopontine and corticobulbar tracts of the ventral pons. He is effectively 'locked in'.

4, J The dilated left pupil was due to a third nerve palsy after the large extradural bleed caused left-sided uncal herniation. The description of extensor posturing is typical of decerebrate posturing and rigidity, suggestive of bilateral midbrain lesions.

5, I The description of the eye movement abnormality is that of internuclear opthalmoplegia (INO)

due to a lesion of the medial longitudinal fasiculus (MLF) which 'yokes' together the ipsilateral III nerve nucleus with the contralateral IV. The rest of the neurology presented suggests a right-sided optic neuritis with cerebellar signs and a previous history of spastic paraparesis. This is suggestive of an INO in the context of multiple sclerosis.

6, K A story of rising blood pressure and a concomitant bradycardia is highly suggestive of compression of the medulla ('coning'). The new neurological signs were presumably a unilateral dilated pupil due to uncal herniation secondary to raised intracranial pressure.

7, C Most acute headaches during intercourse are completely benign but often a subarachnoid haemorrhage may require exclusion. The history given is classical for the latter and this man would require immediate CT brain scan followed by lumbar puncture (looking for xanthochromia) if the scan was normal.

8, D This woman has several risk factors for a cerebral venous sinus thrombosis including probable dehydration secondary to her illegal passage and recent childbirth. Presentation with confusion, headache and seizures is common.

9, A An extradural haemorrhage is suggested from the immediate drop in conscious level and the associated skull fracture. The vessel involved may well be the middle meningeal from the history of temporal skull fracture.

A Follicular thyroid carcinoma
B Oat-cell carcinoma of the lung
C Cushing's disease
D Nelson's syndrome
E Addison's disease
F Primary hyperparathyroidism
G Secondary hyperparathyroidism
H Adrenal cortical tumour
I Adrenal tuberculosis
J Congenital adrenal hyperplasia
K Phaeochromocytoma

For each patient below choose the **SINGLE** most likely diagnosis from the above list of options. Each option may be used once, more than once or not at all.

1 A feature of multiple endocrine neoplasia (MEN) 1 but not multiple endocrine neoplasia (MEN) 2.

2 A feature of MEN 2 but not MEN 1.

3 A feature of both MEN 1 and MEN 2.

4 A 45-year-old male complains of severe weakness. He appears chronically wasted and is mildly hyperpigmented. His blood pressure is 160/100 mmHg. Initial investigations reveal: sodium 142 mmol/l, potassium 3.0 mmol/l, bicarbonate 35 mmol/l, glucose 14 mmol/l. Cortisol levels are 700 nM and are not suppressed by 2 mg dexamethasone every 6 h even after 48 h.

5 A 26-year-old female complains of irregular menses, obesity and low back pain. She has mild hypertension, central obesity, broad striae, acne and mild hirsutism. Initial investigations reveal: sodium 142 mmol/l, potassium 3.9 mmol/l, bicarbonate 25 mmol/l, glucose 12 mmol/l. Cortisol levels are 700 nM before and after 0.5 mg dexamethasone every 6 h, but fall to 300 nM after 2 mg of dexamethasone.

6 A 20-year-old female complains of weakness, easy bruising, hirsutism and irregular menses. She exhibits a moon face, central obesity and severe hirsutism involving the face and trunk, but no virilism. Laboratory values reveal: sodium 142 mmol/l, potassium 3.5 mmol/l, bicarbonate 30 mmol/l, glucose 14 mmol/l. Cortisol levels are 700 nM and are not suppressed by 2 mg dexamethasone every 6 h even after 48 h.

7 A 15-year-old male complains of short stature. He has a history of early sexual development and accelerated growth that ceased 5 years ago. He displays hyperpigmentation. Initial investigations: sodium 139 mmol/l, potassium 4.8 mmol/l, bicarbonate 23 mmol/l, glucose 4.0 mmol/l.

8 Which of the above is associated with reduced pigmentation?

9 A 45-year-old male complains of palpitations. Examination reveals hypertension, and a tachycardia of 120 bpm.

10 A 45-year-old female complains of tingling in her fingers. Plasma vitamin D levels are undetectable.

1, C

2, K

3, F
MEN1 includes primary parathyroid adenomas, pituitary adenomas (Cushing's, acromegaly and prolactinomas) and pancreatic tumours that secrete hormones (insulinomas, glucogonomas, gastrinomas and VIPomas).

MEN2 includes medullary thyroid carcinoma (MTC that secretes calcitonin), phaeochromocytomas and primary parathyroid adenomas.

4, B This is Cushing's syndrome caused by ectopic ACTH.

5, C Cortisol levels classically fall to less than 50% of basal levels after high dose dexamethasone in patients with pituitary dependent Cushing's disease.

6, H This is Cushing's syndrome caused by an adrenal tumour.

7, J Patients with congenital adrenal hyperplasia (CAH) are hyperpigmented because cortisol deficiency causes a high ACTH. When young, excess androgens cause rapid growth and they are initially tall compared to their friends. However, epiphyses then fuse early resulting in final height being short.

8, H An adrenal tumour secreting cortisol will suppress ACTH. The others will either have no effect or a high ACTH.

9, K Phaeochromocytomas secrete catecholamines, responsible for these features.

10, G Low vitamin D levels cause a fall in calcium, which then results in secondary hyperparathyroidism.

A Freidreich's ataxia
B Spinocerebellar ataxia type 2
C Huntington's disease
D Mitochondrial disorder
E Benign intracranial hypertension
F Sagittal venous sinus thrombosis
G Optic nerve sheath glioma
H Neurosarcoidosis
I Cerebellar metastases
J Paraneoplastic cerebellar disorder
K Tobacco–alcohol ambylopia
L Neurosyphilis

For each patient below choose the **SINGLE** most likely match from the above list of options. Each option may be used once, more than once or not at all.

1 A 40-year-old female presents to a psychiatrist with new onset paranoid ideation. Neurological examination including fundoscopy was normal.

2 A 35-year-old male is reviewed in a neurology outpatient clinic. His problems began at the age of 18 with an unsteady gait. Over the years he had increasing difficulty in walking and had been wheel chair bound for the last seven years. At the age of 28 he had become progressively deaf. There was a family history with his maternal grandmother having been diagnosed with progressive myoclonic epilepsy, his maternal aunt with a cerebellar disorder and his mother with deafness.

3 A 41-year-old West Indian male presents with progressive visual failure. He was a heavy drinker and smoker. Fundoscopy showed bilateral papilloedema with visual acuities reduced to hand movement bilaterally only. He had positive syphilis serology on blood testing. MRI/MRV brain imaging was normal. Lumbar puncture showed normal cell count, glucose and protein, with a raised opening pressure.

4 A 42-year-old female presents with new onset cerebellar signs. She had had breast cancer 10 years previously and had been discharged from oncological follow-up five years ago. Her last mammogram had been normal. CT brain was normal.

5 A 60-year-old male presents with unsteady gait. Examination showed papilloedema and nystagmus on looking left or right. There was bilateral finger–nose ataxia, dysdiadochokinesis and dysmetria. He was a heavy smoker and had recently noted blood in his stool.

6 A 60-year-old African female presents with a year-long history of increasing confusion and coarsening of personality. Neuroimaging and lumbar puncture were normal.

1, C A number of neurological conditions can present with an initial psychiatric diagnosis. The age of onset in this woman would be typical of Huntington's disease. However, as we are not given information on the tempo of the disorder, it would be important to consider a metabolic, infective or inflammatory aetiology. Neurosarcoidosis causing an inflammatory CSF process could present in this manner, as could a venous sinus thrombosis. However, the lack of any neurological findings, including papilloedema, make these latter two options less likely.

2, D The history is of an inherited cerebellar ataxia with deafness. The age of onset is most typical of a recessive genetic disorder, making a spinocerebellar ataxia (all autosomal dominant) unlikely. The only two disorders in the list above giving deafness are mitochondrial disorder or Freidreich's ataxia. Mitochondrial disease is the likely diagnosis on the grounds of the matrilineal inheritance pattern (mitochondrial DNA is inherited from the mother) and the history of progressive myoclonic epilepsy in the grandmother [MERRF (myoclonic epilepsy with ragged red fibres) is a mitochondrial disorder].

3, E The history of excess alcohol and tobacco intake would make an amblyopia possible but one would not expect papilloedema. The positive syphilis serology is probably a 'red herring' as many patients of West Indian origin have been exposed to other spirochaete infections, e.g. yaws or pinta, which also give 'positive' syphilis serology. Although neurosyphilis is the 'great mimic' with protean manifestations, this is an unlikely diagnosis, especially in view of the normal CSF cell count. Neurosarcoidosis causing a venous sinus thrombosis or a venous sinus thrombosis *per se* could both give severe papilloedema and eventual visual failure secondary to chronically raised intracranial pressure. The normal MRV and CSF parameters make this less likely. Optic nerve sheath glioma could cause progressive visual failure and papilloedema due to decreased axoplasmic flow along the optic nerve, but would show up on the neuroimaging. Benign intracranial hypertension, although far commoner in females, also occurs in males and is far from benign.

4, J Breast cancer is well known to recur many years after apparent clinical remission. Cerebellar problems could be due either to a cerebellar metastasis from breast cancer or to an autoimmune paraneoplastic condition associated with breast and ovarian malignancies. The normal CT brain makes significant cerebellar metastases less likely. CT brain can be normal in paraneoplastic cerebellar syndromes; MRI brain can sometimes show increased enhancement. An antigen in the tumour is thought to mimic similar epitopes present on cerebellar Purkinje cells (anti-Yo).

5, I The presentation with papilloedema and cerebellar signs is suggestive of cerebellar metastasis either from a chest or bowel primary. The raised intracranial pressure is due to compression of the fourth ventricle and presents a potential neurosurgical emergency.

6, C The length of time since onset of confusion may also be compatible with both neurosyphilis and neurosarcoidosis. However, the normal neuroimaging and lumbar puncture make both of these possibilities unlikely.

A Graves' disease
B Multinodular goitre
C De Quervain's thyroiditis
D Follicular thyroid carcinoma
E Medullary thyroid carcinoma
F Primary hypothyroidism
G Toxic hot nodule
H Primary hypoparathyroidism
I Pseudohypoparathyroidism
J Pseudo-pseudohypoparathyroidism
K Primary hyperparathyroidism

For each patient below choose the **SINGLE** most likely diagnosis from the above list of options. Each option may be used once, more than once or not at all.

1 A 50-year-old female presents with tiredness and is found to have a raised TSH.

2 A 60-year-old female presents with a two-week history of tachycardia and palpitations and is found to have an undetectable TSH. Examination of the eyes reveals lid-lag. A thyroid uptake scan reveals no uptake.

3 A 60-year-old female presents with a two-week history of tachycardia and palpitations and is found to have an undetectable TSH. Examination of the eyes reveals lid-lag. A thyroid uptake scan reveals homogeneous increased uptake.

4 A 50-year-old female presents with a lump in her neck. On direct questioning she admits to severe diarrhoea for the last six months. Her TSH is normal but a thyroid uptake scan reveals a cold nodule.

5 A 6-year-old boy is admitted with a *grand mal* seizure. He is Chvostek's positive. Examination of his hand reveals a short 4th metacarpal.

6 A 40-year-old female complains of constipation. She has a calcium level of 2.72 mmol/l with a normal plasma PTH concentration.

7 A feature of MEN-1.

8 Radioiodine is the usual first line treatment.

9 Patients usually are offered an 18-month course of carbimazole.

10 Thyroidectomy is the first line treatment of choice, followed by radioiodine.

1, F

2, C
De Quervain's thyroiditis (also known as viral thyroiditis) presents with neck pain and dysphagia. This is a viral infection, and the virus causes the thyroid cells to produce more virus instead of taking up iodine. Thus uptake falls immediately. Much stored thyroxine is released by the virally damaged follicles, so the patients present with hyperthyroidism.

3, A   Homogeneous uptake occurs because the entire gland is stimulated by antibodies to the TSH receptor.

4, E   Calcitonin is secreted by medullary thyroid carcinomas and is well known to cause diarrhoea.

5, I   The seizure and Chvostek's sign are present because of hypocalcaemia. The short 4th metacarpal suggests pseudohypoparathyroidism. If the calcium were normal, then pseudo-pseudohypoparathyroidism (J) would be the correct option.

6, K

7, K

8, G

9, A

10, D
Patients given radioiodine before they have any other treatment may be rendered euthyroid, as the labelled iodine is only taken up by the adenoma. This should of course only be undertaken once a malignancy has been excluded by a fine needle aspirate. The adenoma is then suppressed by the radiation, but the normal thyroid (which is inactive, as the TSH is undetectable) does not take up radiation. Once the nodule disappears, the excess thyroxine falls and the TSH rises, stimulating the normal thyroid back into activity. The first line treatment for thyroid cancer is surgery and the first line treatment for Graves' disease is medical treatment with either carbimazole or propylthiouracil.

A   Frontal lobe seizures
B   Simple partial seizures
C   Secondary generalized tonic–clonic seizures
D   Non-epileptic seizures
E   Myoclonic jerks
F   REM sleep related parasomnia
G   Syncopal episodes
H   Stokes–Adams attack
I   Petit mal epilepsy
J   Grand mal epilepsy
K   Temporal lobe epilepsy
L   Absence epilepsy

For each patient below choose the **SINGLE** most likely match from the above list of options. Each option may be used once, more than once or not at all.

1   A 20-year-old male gives a five-year history of seizures. These occur solely at night, often between 04.00 and 06.00 hours. During these episodes he is often incontinent and occasionally bites his tongue. The attacks are frequent, up to five a night.

2   A 20-year-old male gives a five-year history of blank episodes. His partner describes these as often occurring whilst he is talking. He stops talking and makes a groaning noise. He makes lip-smacking noises and swallowing motions. His right hand is clenched in a fist. His left hand often pulls at the buttons of his shirt.

3   A 32-year-old woman had a head injury a year earlier following a road traffic accident. She gives a two-month history of sudden onset cold sensations along her left arm and left side of her face.

These last for a few seconds only. They can occur up to 10 times a day.

4   A 15-year-old male presents with headache and papilloedema. He gives a recent history of jerking of the fingers of his right hand. The jerking does not spread up the arm and lasts for a couple of minutes at a time.

5   A 50-year-old male gives a three-month history of seizures. He has no warning to these episodes and remembers nothing about them. His wife describes him falling to the floor and shaking his arms and legs for two to three minutes. He occasionally bites his tongue and is often incontinent of urine.

6   An 18-year-old female presents with new onset seizures. She sometimes has a warning that something is about to happen. She then falls to the floor and is aware of jerking movements of her arms and legs. Her back and neck often arch during these attacks. She is often incontinent of urine and sometimes bites the inside of her cheek.

7   A 22-year-old male presents with blackouts. He describes six attacks over the last three months. He describes feeling clammy and sweaty before losing consciousness. A routine electroencephalogram (EEG), 24-h cardiac tape and CT brain scan were normal.

8   An 80-year-old male has blackouts. He feels his heart racing prior to these and his wife describes him as appearing like a ghost when he is unconscious. During one of these episodes he was noted to have twitching movements of his arms and legs lasting seconds only.

1, A   The history of frequent, purely nocturnal seizures is highly suggestive of frontal lobe epilepsy. Bizarre movements are observed during these seizures including 'bicycling' movements of the legs.

2, K   The description is typical for complex partial seizures of temporal lobe origin. The dystonic posturing of the right hand suggests a left temporal lobe ictal focus, which is further supported by the automatisms of the ipsilateral hand. Lip-smacking is again typical of temporal lobe epilepsy (TLE).

3, B   The description of unilateral fleeting sensory symptoms after head injury would be compatible with partial seizures with an ictal focus in the contra-lateral sensory strip of the parietal lobe.

4, E   The presentation with headache and papilloedema is suggestive of an intracranial mass lesion. The subsequent description of jerking of the fingers of the right hand would be compatible with either a motor partial seizure or myoclonic jerking. The lack of a Jacksonian march, with seizure spread from the fingers proceeding proximally up the arm, is more suggestive of myoclonus.

Both myoclonus and partial seizures can be secondary to a mass lesion in the contralateral parietal lobe.

5, J   The description is compatible with tonic–clonic seizures. There is no aura to suggest secondary generalization.

6, D   There is no loss of awareness during this generalized seizure making epilepsy unlikely. Back arching is also highly suggestive of non-epileptic seizures. Urinary incontinence is not pathognomonic for epilepsy.

7, G   The description of feeling sweaty or clammy before passing out is suggestive of a syncopal event. The normal 24-h tape suggests no associated arrythmia. Tunnel vision prior to blacking out may also be described.

8, H   Stokes–Adams attacks are cardiac arrythmia associated with loss of consciousness. The classical description is of the patient appearing white, with the blood drained from their face. The description of twitching of the limbs during the attack may well be an anoxia related tonic–clonic seizure as a secondary event.

A Diabetic ketoacidosis
B Hyperosmolar non-ketotic coma
C Hypoglycaemia
D Hyperglycaemia
E Hypercalcaemia with calcium 2.75
F Hypocalcaemia with calcium 2.03
G Respiratory alkalosis
H Respiratory acidosis
I Compensated respiratory acidosis
J Hyponatraemia
K Hypokalaemia

For each patient below choose the **SINGLE** most likely diagnosis from the above list of options. Each option may be used once, more than once or not at all.

1 A 22-year-old female presents with carpal spasm. She complains that she feels very breathless, and that attacks of severe breathlessness and carpal spasm have occurred about once a week, since her boyfriend left her.

2 A 14-year-old female complains of thirst and polyuria for the last three days, with nocturia for the last three nights. She complains that she feels breathless.

3 A 65-year-old male presents unconscious to casualty. He has been complaining of nocturia for

the last two years. Examination reveals severe dehydration. Initial electrolytes reveal sodium 169 mmol/l.

4 A 25-year-old male presents unconscious to casualty. He is a known type 1 diabetic. He is unrousable and examination reveals a tachycardia and hypertension.

5 A 50-year-old male is found to have an adrenal tumour when investigated for hypertension.

6 A 65-year-old male presents unconscious to casualty. Initial electrolytes reveal: sodium 145 mmol/l, potassium 3.9 mmol/l, bicarbonate 42 mmol/l.

7 A 60-year-old male presents with the following arterial blood gases: pH 7.39, $pCO_2 = 9$ kPa, $pO_2 = 5$ kPa.

8 A 25-year-old female presents with a significant overdose of aspirin.

9 A 25-year-old male presents unconscious to casualty. He has taken an overdose of temazepam and heroin, both intravenously.

10 A 45-year-old male presents unconscious to casualty. He has taken an overdose of chlorpropamide.

1, G Hyperventilation causes a fall in carbon dioxide, and hence an alkalosis.

2, A

3, B

4, C

5, K
Hypertension associated with an adrenal tumour is caused by either excess cortisol (Cushing's syndrome), excess aldosterone (Conn's syndrome) or excess catecholamines (phaeochromocytoma). All will cause hypokalaemia.

6, I This patient will have been compensating for a respiratory acidosis for some time by retaining bicarbonate.

7, I This is likely to be the same patient as in (6), but this time you get the gas results back first.

8, G Aspirin is a primary respiratory stimulant, and can cause a respiratory alkalosis as a result. A metabolic acidosis can also occur as salicylate is itself an acid.

9, H This combination is a potent respiratory suppressant; thus, carbon dioxide levels rise.

10, C

A   Multiple systems atrophy
B   Idiopathic Parkinson's disease
C   Wilson's disease
D   Huntington's chorea
E   Hyperthyroidism
F   Progressive supranuclear palsy (Steele-Richardson–Olsewski syndrome)
G   Normal pressure hydrocephalus
H   Niemann–Pick type C disease
I   Diffuse Lewy body disease
J   McArdle's disease
K   Amyotrophic lateral sclerosis

For each patient below choose the **SINGLE** most likely match from the above list of options. Each option may be used once, more than once or not at all.

1   A 60-year-old male presents with falls and difficulty in reading, problems in walking down stairs and difficulty in co-ordinating lighting his cigarette with a match.

2   A 13-year-old female presents with behavioural problems at home and school. Examination reveals a coarse tremor of both out-stretched arms and slurring of speech.

3   A 75-year-old female presents with confusion, change in personality and gradual memory loss. Examination reveals a postural drop in systolic blood pressure of 30 mmHg, a score of 20/30 on the mini-mental test score, bilateral cogwheeling rigidity and impaired postural reflexes.

4   A 65-year-old female is examined in an opthamology clinic. She has a visual acuity of 6/6 bilaterally corrected with glasses. Fundoscopy is normal. Examination of pursuit and voluntary paced saccades shows reduced upgaze and downgaze. This deficit corrects on oculo-cephalic reflex testing.

5   A 25-year-old female presents with agitation and fidgety movements. There is no family history of note. Examination reveals bilateral chorea of the upper limbs. All routine blood tests are normal.

6   A 20-year-old male presents with a one-year history of slowing up of his walking. He had become aware of a change in his handwriting, which was increasingly unrecognizable. Examination revealed a festinant gait, impaired postural reflexes, difficulty in turning, four limb rigidity and decreased amplitude of movements.

He had facial hypomimia. There was no family history of neurological disease. His mother was alive and well but his father had committed suicide in his late forties.

7   A 68-year-old female gave a four-year history of impaired gait, falls, urinary frequency and incontinence. Examination revealed upper limb rigidity with decreased amplitude of movement. There was bilateral finger–nose ataxia, dysdiadochokinesis, heel–toe and heel–shin ataxia. Anal sphincter electromyograph was markedly abnormal.

8   A 68-year-old female presented with falls and a tremor first noted by her family. Examination revealed facial hypomimia, a positive glabellar tap and a rest tremor of the right hand. She had cogwheeling rigidity, more marked on the right-hand side, and reduction in amplitude of movement with bradykinesia. She had a postural drop of 30 mmHg systolic on standing. She was referred for sphincter EMG, which was mildly abnormal. Three months prior to being seen, she had begun to develop florid hallucinations.

9   A 20-year-old Indian female was brought to the UK for a private neurology opinion. Her parents gave a six-year history of problems beginning with abnormal movements of both arms noticed by the family. On occasions her right hand would adopt a fist-like posture. She began to perform badly in her college work and eventually had to be removed from college. Her younger brother had had similar problems and had died at the age of 14.

10   A 68-year-old male came to a neurology outpatient clinic for his yearly review. He had been diagnosed with idiopathic Parkinson's disease two years previously. He was on a combination of benzhexol and cabergoline, which had been recently started. He complained of increasing falls and dizzy spells. Examination revealed parkinsonism and a postural drop of 30 mmHg systolic.

11   A 14-year-old Pakistani female was brought to clinic for an opinion. Her parents gave a three-year history of progressive cognitive decline such that her mental age was now equivalent to her 8-year-old brother. They had noted a progressive deterioration in her gait and a tendency for her feet to turn inwards on walking. Examination revealed a supranuclear gaze palsy with marked parkinsonism and dystonia of both upper and lower limbs.

1, F The history of early falls is suggestive of an extra-pyramidal problem causing loss of postural reflexes. The difficulty in reading a book, walking downstairs and lighting a match is due to a supranuclear gaze palsy causing problems in looking down. Progressive supranuclear gaze palsy is the combination of a supranuclear gaze palsy together with akinetic rigidity.

2, C This young woman has presented with behavioural problems together with a tremor and cerebellar speech. The likeliest underlying cause from the list is Wilson's disease, which can present with a predominant psychiatric phenotype and various types of tremor, including cerebellar and a characteristic 'wing-beating' tremor.

3, I This elderly woman has presented with dementia, extrapyramidal features and a significant postural drop. The postural drop is suggestive of underlying autonomic problems: these may occur in multiple systems atrophy (MSA), however, significant dementia is uncommon in this condition. The likely diagnosis is thus diffuse Lewy body disease, which can cause autonomic problems due to Lewy body formation in the autonomic ganglia.

4, F This woman has a supranuclear gaze palsy with difficulty in vertical gaze. This is correctable on oculo-cephalic testing confirming the integrity of the lower motor nuclei. The likely diagnosis is PSP.

5, D This young woman has presented with chorea. Despite the lack of a family history, sporadic Huntington's chorea is still possible. However, other causes of chorea need to be excluded including hyperthyroidism, polycythaemia rubra vera and systemic lupus. The normal blood tests exclude the latter causes.

6, D This young man has presented with parkinsonism. There is no family history of neurological disease, however, the history of his father committing suicide may be relevant in this clinical setting. Patients without overt features of Huntington's disease have been known to commit suicide: this may be related to the psychiatric/behavioural features of the disease or due to retention of insight into emerging neurological problems. This man has the Westphal version of Huntington's with presentation in youth with a parkinsonian picture.

7, A This elderly woman has given a history of parkinsonism, sphincter disturbance and cerebellar signs. The likeliest diagnosis is MSA cerebellar type (type C).

8, I This woman has presented with parkinsonism together with a significant postural drop. Sphincter EMG is used in the diagnosis of MSA and is highly reliable. However, abnormalities have also been reported in normals, especially multiparous females. Hallucinations are typical in the presentation of diffuse Lewy body disease.

9, C This young woman has presented with involuntary movements first noticed by her family. These include dystonic posturing of the right hand. There is a suggestion of cognitive decline with her deteriorating college work. There is a family history with her brother affected. This would all be compatible with an underlying diagnosis of Wilson's disease.

10, B This elderly man initially presented with apparent idiopathic Parkinson's disease. He has then developed a significant postural drop after initiation of cabergoline treatment. Cabergoline is a long-acting dopamine agonist and has side-effects including significant postural hypotension.

11, H This young woman has presented with parkinsonism, cognitive decline, limb dystonia and a supranuclear gaze palsy. All of these features are seen in Niemann–Pick type C. Niemann–Pick types A and B are infantile disorders caused by deficiency of sphingomyelinase. Lysosomal storage of sphingomyelin, cholesterol and glycolipids occurs. Clinical features include organomegaly, a cherry-red spot on fundoscopy and psychomotor retardation. Type C can have a young adult onset and has the additional neurological features outlined above.

A Rheumatic heart disease with aortic and mitral valve stenosis and systemic embolism
B Atrial septal defect and mitral stenosis with thromboembolism
C Ischaemic cardiomyopathy, atrial fibrillation with systemic thromboembolism
D Infective endocarditis with septic embolism
E Left atrial myxoma with systemic embolism

For each patient below choose the **SINGLE** most likely match from the above list of options. Each option may be used once, more than once or not at all.

1 A 62-year-old female is admitted with a one year history of malaise, exertional dyspnoea but no orthopnoea or paroxysmal nocturnal dyspnoea. She had developed a painful left leg with subsequent numbness one week previously. There was a history of childhood rheumatic fever. On examination, her pulse was 120/min, irregularly irregular with an audible ejection systolic murmur at the right upper sternal edge and a mid-diastolic murmur at the apex. The left foot pulses were absent. Her initial investigations were as follows:
ECG: atrial fibrillation, right bundle branch block, right axis deviation
Chest X-ray: cardiomegaly, an increased angle at the carina

2 A 50-year-old male is admitted with a one year history of exertional chest pain and dyspnoea and orthopnoea. He had developed weakness of his right arm and leg two days previously. There was a history of previous anterior myocardial infarction, hypertension and smoking. On examination, his pulse was 120/min, irregularly irregular with a blood pressure of 180/100. There was mild weakness of his right side with an extensor plantar response. The initial investigations were as follows:
ECG: atrial fibrillation, voltage criteria for left ventricular hypertrophy
Chest X-ray: cardiomegaly

3 A 62-year-old female is admitted with a two-month history of malaise, sweats and exertional dyspnoea. She had developed expressive dysphasia on the day of admission. There was a history of childhood rheumatic fever. On examination, her pulse was 120/min, irregularly irregular with an audible ejection systolic murmur at the left upper sternal edge and a mid-diastolic murmur at the apex. Her initial investigations were as follows:
ECG: atrial fibrillation
Chest X-ray: cardiomegaly, an increased angle at the carina
Haematology: Hb 9 g/dl, WCC 18×10^9/l, Plts 200×10^9/l, urea 14.1 mmol/l, creatinine 250 μmol/l, ESR 100 mm/h
Urinalysis: haematuria

4 A 60-year-old woman is admitted with a years history of malaise, exertional dyspnoea and orthopnoea. She had developed a painful left leg with subsequent numbness one week previously. There was a history of childhood rheumatic fever. On examination, her pulse was 120/min, irregularly irregular with an audible ejection systolic murmur at the left upper sternal edge and a mid-diastolic murmur at the apex. The left foot pulses were absent. Her initial investigations were as follows:
ECG: atrial fibrillation
Chest X-ray: cardiomegaly, an increased angle at the carina
ESR 20 mm/h

5 A 56-year-old female presents with a one-year history of exertional dyspnoea, fever and weight loss. On examination the pulse was 120/min, irregularly irregular with an audible mid-diastolic murmur at the apex. Her initial investigations were as follows:
ESR 80 mm/h
ECG: atrial fibrillation
Chest X-ray: normal
Hb 9 g/dl, WCC 8×10^9/l, Plts 200×10^9/l

1, B A history of exertional dyspnoea in the absence of orthopnoea and paroxysmal nocturnal dyspnoea is characteristic of Lutembacher's syndrome. This is the rare association of mitral stenosis with a secundum atrial septal defect. The ECG findings are consistent with those of a secundum atrial septal defect. The thromboembolic episode may be secondary to the presence of mitral stenosis, atrial fibrillation or the atrial septal defect (paradoxical embolism).

2, C This man has presented with ischaemic heart disease and hypertension. His history would be consistent with left ventricular impairment, secondary to previous myocardial infarction, poorly controlled hypertension with a further possible contribution from his existing ischaemic heart disease (anginal equivalent dyspnoea). The thromboembolic episode may have been consequent to atrial fibrillation or left ventricular dilatation and systolic impairment.

3, D The history and physical findings would support a diagnosis of valvular heart disease and infective endocarditis. This is further supported by an elevated ESR, renal impairment and haematuria.

4, A This woman's history of childhood rheumatic fever, together with her clinical signs, makes rheumatic valve disease, with atrial fibrillation and systemic embolism the most likely possibility. Risk factors for systemic embolism in mitral stenosis include: older age; increased size of left atrial appendage; atrial fibrillation and low cardiac output. Atrial fibrillation is present in 80% of patients who embolize. Cerebral emboli constitute 50% of emboli.

5, E Myxomas are the commonest primary cardiac tumour. The commonest site is the left atrium (86% cases). They may present with non-specific features or may present following embolism or due to mechanical interference with valvular function (the mitral valve in this case). The symptoms may be intermittent, sudden in onset and affected by body position. Atrial fibrillation, an elevated ESR and anaemia are documented associations.

Listing by specialty

Question number:

Audiometry medicine	97
Cardiology	1, 4, 7, 9, 12, 14, 16, 19, 22, 24, 27, 30, 34, 36, 38, 41, 44, 46, 49, 52, 55, 59, 61, 64, 67, 71, 74, 78, 90, 85, 83, 85, 90, 92, , 96, 100, EMQ 8
Chemical pathology	17, 42, 51, 72, 84
Endocrinology	6, 10, 18, 25, 33, 62, 81, 86, 95, 99, EMQ 2, EMQ 4, EMQ 6
Gastroenterology	5, 11, 15, 21, 26, 27, 40, 66, 77, 87, 93, 101
Genetics	69
Haematology	2, 13, 23, 32, 39, 50, 75, 88, 91
Infectious diseases	3, 35, 43, 45, 48, 57, 63, 70, 79, 94
Neurology	76, EMQ 1, EMQ 3, EMQ 5, EMQ 7
Oncology	8
Psychiatry	82
Renal medicine	28, 31, 54, 58, 73
Respiratory medicine	20, 37, 47, 53, 56, 60, 89, 98
Rheumatology	65, 68

Index

Numbers are page numbers, not question numbers. Page numbers in *italics* refer to figures.

abdominal pain 187, 188
ACTH *see* adrenocorticotrophic hormone
activated protein C resistance 4
acute renal failure
    analgesic-induced 107, 108
    on chronic 38
    postoperative 55, 56
Addisonian crisis 49, 50
adenosine 24
ADH *see* antidiuretic hormone
adrenalectomy, bilateral total 49, 50, 197, 198
adrenal infarction 158
adrenal insufficiency
    in AIDS 90
    iatrogenic primary 49, 50
    in meningococcal sepsis 157, 158
adrenalitis 90
adrenocorticotrophic hormone (ACTH)
    ectopic secretion 123, 124
    hypersecretion 50, 198
adult respiratory distress syndrome *195*, 196
AIDS/HIV infection
    abdominal pain 187, 188
    autoimmune thrombocytopaenia 175, 176
    cryptococcal meningitis 69, 70
    macrocytosis 181, 182
    seizures 5, 6, 89, 90
alcoholic liver disease 9, 10, 185, 186
alkalosis, metabolic *see* metabolic alkalosis
allopurinol 100
alpha-fetoprotein, serum 41, 42
alveolitis, fibrosing 93, 94
amenorrhoea 189, 190
aminoglycoside therapy 152
amiodarone-induced hypothyroidism 35, 36
amyloidosis, secondary 136
anaemia
    breathlessness 119, 120
    drug-induced haemolytic 149, 150
    leukoerythroblastic 15, 16
    macrocytic *see* macrocytosis
    mechanical valve haemolysis 7, 8
    pernicious 46

analgesic-induced interstitial nephritis 107, 108
anorexia (nervosa) 77, 78
antibiotic prophylaxis 179, 180
anticonvulsant (antiepileptic) drugs 45, 46, 83, 84
antidiuretic hormone (ADH)
    deficiency 168
    syndrome of inappropriate secretion (SIADH) 90, 162
antihypertensive drugs 149, 150, 159, 160
antiphospholipid antibodies 4
antipsychotic drugs 163, 164
aorta, coarctation of 179, 180
aortic regurgitation *133*, 134
aortic stenosis
    mild 1, 2
    moderate 103, 104
    severe rheumatic 117, 118
aortic valve
    area 118
    bicuspid *75*, 76
    gradient 117, 118
    replacement 35, 91
arterio-venous malformation, pulmonary 177, 178
arthritis
    gonococcal 139, 140
    rheumatoid 135, 136
asthma
    eosinophilia and 105, 106
    flow-volume loops *73*, 74
    respiratory failure 111, 112
asymmetrical septal hypertrophy (ASH) *109*, 110, 156
atelectasis, bilateral pulmonary 183, 184
atrial bigemini *17*, 18
atrial ectopic beats *17*, 18
atrial fibrillation *191*, 192
    in haemochromatosis 79
    with slow ventricular response 31, 32
atrial flutter
    with 2:1 block *23*, 24, 43
    with ventricular tachycardia *43*, 44

atrial septal defect, repaired 71, 72
atrioventricular block
    atrial flutter with *23*, 24, 43
    first degree *37*, 38, *169*, 170
    Mobitz type II second degree *165*, 166
    third degree (complete) *27*, 28, 166
atrioventricular bypass tracts 48
audiogram *193*, 194
auditory meatus, obstruction 194
Austin–Flint murmur 133, 134
autoimmune disease, primary biliary cirrhosis
    association 58
automatic implantable cardioverter-defibrillator
    (AICD) 199, 200
azathioprine 99, 100

back pain
    chronic 107, 108
    leukoerythroblastic anaemia with 15, 16
    osteoporosis 63, 64
bacterial endocarditis *see* infective endocarditis
Bartter's syndrome 61, 62
bendrofluazide 13, 14
β-adrenoceptor blocker 159, 160
biliary obstruction, prolonged 174
biliary stent, blocked 29, 30
blood transfusion, past history 153
bone marrow metastases 16
bradycardia
    in hypothermia *53*, 54
    sinus *159*, 160
bromocriptine 190
bronchial carcinoma 122
    dermatomyositis and 129, 130
    oat cell 124
bronze diabetes 80
bulimia 62
burr cells 185, 186

cabergoline 190
caeruloplasmin, decreased levels 173, 174
caffeine 18
calcium gluconate 38
carbon monoxide
    corrected transfer (KCO) 119, 120
    diffusing factor (D$_L$CO) 119, 120

transfer factor (T$_L$CO) 39, 119, 120
cardiac failure
    biventricular 1
    congestive 71, 72
    end-stage 37, 38
cardiomyopathy, hypertrophic *see* hypertrophic
    (obstructive) cardiomyopathy
cardioverter-defibrillator, automatic implantable
    (AICD) 199, 200
cerebral infarction 127, 128
cerebral malaria 86
cerebrospinal fluid (CSF) rhinorrhoea 125, 126
chest infections, recurrent 67, 68
chest pain
    exertional 1
    intermittent 143
    severe central 101, 102
chicken-pox pneumonitis 195, 196
cholangiocarcinoma 29, 30
cholangitis, ascending 29, 30
cholestasis, familial intrahepatic 174
cholesterol, elevated 101, 102
chronic active hepatitis, autoimmune 153, 154
chronic obstructive airways disease (COAD) 74
Churg–Strauss syndrome 105, 106
cimetidine 116, 187, 188
cirrhosis, primary biliary (PBC) 57, 58, 174
clotting abnormality 171, 172
clubbing
    and cyanosis 93, 94
    and haemoptysis 121, 122
    in Kartagener's syndrome 67, 68
CMV *see* cytomegalovirus
coarctation of aorta 179, 180
coeliac disease 131, 132
coma, hypoglycaemic 85, 86
conducting system disease, diffuse *165*, 166
continuity equation 118
Coombs' test 150
co-trimoxazole, adverse effects 90
creatine kinase (CK), elevated 163, 164
creatinine, elevated urinary 115, 116
Crigler–Najjar type II syndrome 52
cryoglobulinaemia, essential 146
cryptococcal meningitis 69, 70
CSF rhinorrhoea 125, 126
Cushing's disease, past history 49, 50, 197,
    198

Cushing's syndrome 123, 124
cyanosis, and clubbing 93, 94
cytomegalovirus (CMV)
    adrenalitis 90
    encephalitis 6, 70, 90
cytotoxic agent therapy 58

deafness, unilateral conduction *193*, 194
death, sudden 156
delta agent infection 114
dermatomyositis 129, 130
dexamethasone test, high dose 124
dextrocardia *67*, 68
diabetes, bronze 80
diabetes insipidus 168
diabetic ketoacidosis 11, 12
diarrhoea, offensive 171, 172
didanosine (DDI) 187, 188
digitalis/digoxin
    in hypokalaemia 13, 14
    warfarin and 192
diuretics
    abuse 62
    fluid over-infusion with 33, 34
    induced hypokalaemia 13, 14
Dubin–Johnson syndrome 52

ear disease, middle 194
Ebstein's anomaly 48
encephalitis
    Cytomegalovirus (CMV) 6, 70, 90
    Herpes simplex virus (HSV) 6, 70, 90
    HIV 6
    Varicella zoster 6
endocarditis
    infective *see* infective endocarditis
    Liebman–Sacks 127, 128
endotracheal intubation, previous 40, 195, 196
eosinophilia 105, 106
epilepsy
    pancytopaenia 45, 46
    status epilepticus 83, 84
    see also seizures
Epstein–Barr virus (EBV) infection 95, 96
erythema *ab igne* 19
exhaustion, in severe asthma 111, 112

factor V Leiden 4
Felty's syndrome 136
FEV$_1$/FVC ratio 40, 94
fibrosing alveolitis 93, 94
Fitz–Hugh–Curtis syndrome 140
flow-volume loops
    after chicken-pox pneumonitis *195*, 196
    in asthma *73*, 74
fluid therapy
    excessive postoperative 33, 34
    inadequate postoperative 55, 56
folic acid deficiency 46

galactorrhoea 189, 190
gammopathy, benign monoclonal 25, 26
genetic counselling 137, 138
Gilbert's syndrome 51, 52
glandular fever 95, 96
gonococcal arthritis 139, 140
gonorrhoea 140
Goodpasture's syndrome 146
gout 100

haemochromatosis, hereditary 79, 80
haemolysis
    drug-induced autoimmune 149, 150
    mechanical valve 8
haemoptysis
    clubbing and 121, 122
    dermatomyositis and 129, 130
    pleuritic pain with 177, 178
    pulmonary-renal condition with 145, 146
haemosiderinuria 150
haptoglobins, serum 150
headaches
    early morning 167, 168
    galactorrhoea and 189, 190
heart block *see* atrioventricular block
heart failure *see* cardiac failure
heart valves, prosthetic *see* prosthetic heart valves
hemiparesis, left-sided 127, 128
Henoch–Schonlein purpura 146
hepatitis
    autoimmune (lupoid) chronic active 153, 154
    viral 113, 114
hepatitis A 96

hepatitis B 96
  carrier 113, 114
  previous exposure 21, 22
  transmission risk 113, 114
hepatitis C 96, 114
hepatitis E 114
hepatocellular carcinoma, primary 41, 42
Herpes simplex virus (HSV) encephalitis 6, 70, 90
hip fracture 33, 34
HIV
  encephalitis 6
  infection *see* AIDS/HIV infection
  seroconversion illness 96
Howell–Jolly bodies 131, 132
human immunodeficiency virus *see* HIV
hydralazine 144
hyperbilirubinaemia, familial 51, 52
hypercalcaemia 15, 16
hypercholesterolaemia 101, 102
hyperkalaemia
  ECG changes *37*, 38
  postoperative 55, 56
hyperprolactinaemia 189, 190
hypertension, treated 149, 150, 159, 160
hypertrophic (obstructive) cardiomyopathy
  asymmetrical septal hypertrophy *109*, 110
  left ventricular outflow tract gradient *155*, 156
  systolic anterior motion of mitral valve *97*, 98
hypoadrenalism *see* adrenal insufficiency
hypoglycaemic coma 85, 86
hypokalaemia
  Bartter's syndrome 61, 62
  dilutional 33, 34
  ECG changes *13*, 14
hyponatraemia
  in AIDS 89, 90
  dilutional 33, 34
  hypothyroidism 161, 162
hypophosphataemic (vitamin D resistant) rickets
    137, 138
hyposplenism 131, 132
hypothalamic tumour 168
hypothermia
  ECG changes *53*, 54
  primary hypothyroidism 19
hypothyroidism
  amiodarone-induced 35, 36
  autoimmune 58

hyponatraemia 161, 162
  in pituitary/hypothalamic disease 168
  primary 19, 20
  subclinical 65, 66
hypoxia 90

infectious mononucleosis 95, 96
infective endocarditis
  coarctation of aorta risk 179, 180
  intravenous drug abuse 21, 22
  subacute right-sided 146
  transoesophageal echocardiography *141*, 142
intensive therapy unit (ITU), previous admission
    39, 40, 195
interstitial nephritis, acute 107, 108
intracranial pressure, raised 168, 190
intracranial space occupying lesion 90
intravenous drug abuse 21, 22
intravenous fluids *see* fluid therapy
iron
  deficiency 131, 132
  overload 79, 80

jaundice
  alcoholic liver disease 9, 10
  obstructive 29, 30
  viral hepatitis 113, 114
J waves, in hypothermia *53*, 54

kaolin-cephalin clotting time (KCCT) 3, 4
Kartagener's syndrome 67, 68
Kayser–Fleischer rings 174
ketoacidosis, diabetic 11, 12
ketoconazole, adverse effects 90

laxative abuse 62
left atrial pressure, elevated 92
left axis deviation *81*, 82
left bundle branch block *37*, 38
left to right shunt 71, 72
left ventricular end diastolic pressure, elevated 92
left ventricular outflow tract gradient *155*, 156
leukoerythroblastic anaemia 15, 16
libido, decreased 167, 168

Liebman–Sacks endocarditis 127, 128
liquorice overdose 62
liver disease, alcoholic 9, 10, 185, 186
lung
    collapse, segmental 112
    fibrosis 196
lung disease
    obstructive 94
        asthma 73, 74
        tracheal stenosis 39, 40, 196
    restrictive 94, 143, 144, 196
lupus, drug-induced 143, 144
lupus anticoagulant 4, 140
lupus erythematosus, systemic see systemic lupus
        erythematosus

macrocytosis
    in AIDS 181, 182
    alcoholic liver disease 9, 10
    hypothyroidism 20, 161, 162
    primary biliary cirrhosis 57, 58
malabsorption 171, 172
malaria
    cerebral 86
    falciparum 85, 86
malnutrition, severe 77, 78
mechanical valve haemolysis 8
meningitis
    bacterial 125, 126
    cryptococcal 69, 70
    tuberculous 70
meningococcal sepsis 157, 158
metabolic alkalosis
    hypokalaemic 61, 62
    hyponatraemic, hypokalaemic 33, 34
metastases, bone marrow 16
α-methyldopa 150
mitral incompetence 71, 72
mitral stenosis
    critical 1, 2
    mild 59, 60
    severe 147, 148
mitral valve
    area, normal 2
    balloon valvuloplasty 148
    gradient 147, 148
    prolapse 48

replacement 7, 8, 191, 192
    systolic anterior motion (SAM) 97, 98, 110, 156
M-mode echocardiogram
    bicuspid aortic valve 75, 76
    hypertrophic cardiomyopathy 97, 98
    mitral stenosis 59, 60
monoclonal gammopathy of uncertain
        significance (MGUS) 25, 26
muscle
    spasms, painful 131, 132
    twitching 37, 38
myasthenia gravis 151, 152
myeloma, multiple 16, 26, 64
myocardial infarction
    acute 27, 28
    previous 169, 170
myopathy
    drug-induced 101, 102
    proximal 123, 124, 129, 130

Nelson's syndrome 49, 50, 197, 198
neuroleptic malignant syndrome 163, 164

obesity, in hypothyroidism 19, 20
oral contraceptive pill 87, 88
osmolality, plasma 167, 168
osteomalacia 172
osteoporosis 63, 64

pacemaker
    failure 31, 32
    indication 165, 166, 169, 170
pancreatitis 188
pancytopaenia
    in epilepsy 45, 46
    in rheumatoid arthritis 135, 136
parenteral nutrition 77, 78
pericardial effusion 20, 121, 122
pernicious anaemia 46
phenytoin 45, 46
pigmentation, skin 49, 50, 197, 198
pituitary tumour
    ACTH-secreting 50, 198
    diabetes insipidus 167, 168
    prolactin-secreting 189, 190

plasma osmolality 167, 168
Plasmodium falciparum 85, 86
pleural effusion
    bilateral 65, 66
    drug-induced lupus 143
    echocardiography *121*, 122
pleuritic pain 177, 178
Pneumococcus carinii pneumonia (PCP) 89, 90
pneumonitis, chicken-pox 195, 196
pneumothorax 112
polyarteritis nodosa 146
P pulmonale *87*, 88
primary biliary cirrhosis (PBC) 57, 58, 174
procainamide, long-term therapy 143, 144
progressive multifocal leucoencephalopathy 90
prolactinoma 190
prosthetic heart valves
    digitalis and *191*, 192
    dysfunction 91, 92
    mechanical valve haemolysis 7, 8
protein C resistance, activated 4
pulmonary arterio-venous malformation 177, 178
pulmonary atelectasis, bilateral 183, 184
pulmonary embolism
    ECG changes *183*, 184
    recurrent septic 146
    thrombophilia 3, 4
pulmonary haemorrhage 177, 178
pulmonary hypertension 87, 88
pulmonary thromboembolic disease 88
P waves, bifid *81*, *82*, *169*, 170
pyelonephritis 151, 152
pyloric stenosis, chronic 62

quadrantinopia 189, 190
quinagolide 190
quinidine 43, 44
quinine 85, 86

rectal (PR) bleeding 119, 120
renal impairment
    acute *see* acute renal failure
    in alcoholic liver disease 185, 186
    Churg–Strauss syndrome 105, 106
    leukoerythroblastic anaemia and 15, 16
renal transplant patient 99, 100

renal tubular disorder, primary 62
'reversed tick' appearance *191*, 192
re-warming, in hypothermia *53*, 54
rheumatoid arthritis 135, 136
rhinorrhoea, CSF 125, 126
rickets, vitamin D resistant (hypophosphataemic)
        137, 138
right axis deviation *169*, 170
    in Kartagener's syndrome *67*, 68
    mitral valve replacement *191*, 192
    in pulmonary hypertension 87, 88
right bundle branch block *81*, *82*, *169*, 170
    mitral valve replacement *191*, 192
    in pulmonary embolism *183*, 184
right ventricular hypertrophy *87*, 88
Rotor syndrome 52
R waves, reversed progression *67*, 68

schizophrenia 163, 164
seizures
    in HIV infection 5, 6, 89, 90
    see also epilepsy
septal hypertrophy, asymmetrical (ASH) *109*, 110,
        156
shivering, ECG artefacts *53*, 54
simvastatin 102
sinusitis, recurrent 67, 68
sinus node disease *159*, 160
$S_IQ_{III}T_{III}$ pattern *183*, 184
Sjogren's disease 136
skin pigmentation 49, 50, 197, 198
skull fracture, previous 125, 126
SLE *see* systemic lupus erythematosus
small stature
    flow-volume loops *195*, 196
    syndromic 61, 62
space occupying lesion, intracranial 90
splenomegaly, in rheumatoid arthritis 135, 136
splinter haemorrhages 21
status epilepticus 83, 84
steatorrhoea 171, 172
stomach carcinoma 183, 184
stroke (cerebral infarction) 127, 128
ST segment
    depression *13*, 14, *27*, 28
    elevation 27, 28
    sagging *191*, 192

sudden death 156
syndrome of inappropriate antidiuretic hormone
    secretion (SIADH) 90, 162
systemic lupus erythematosus (SLE) 146
    cerebral infarction 127, 128
    lupus anticoagulant 4

tachycardia
    sinus *183*, 184
    ventricular *see* ventricular tachycardia
target cells 10, 185, 186
tetracosactrin test, short 158
theophylline derivatives 18
thiazide diuretics 13, 14
thrombocytopaenia, autoimmune 175, 176
thrombophilia 3, 4
thyroxine replacement therapy 19, 20
tonsillitis, acute 49, 50
toxoplasmosis 70
tracheal stenosis 40, 196
transoesophageal echocardiography *141*, 142,
    148
travellers, returned 85, 86, 113
tricuspid valve endocarditis 22
trifascicular block *169*, 170
trimethoprim 115, 116
tuberculous meningitis 70
T waves
    inverted *183*, 184
    tented *37*, 38

uridyldiphosphate glucuronyl transferase
    (UDPGT), reduced activity 52

urinary tract infection 115, 116
    in myasthenia gravis 151, 152
U waves, prominent *13*, 14

vagotonic manoeuvres 24
valproate, sodium 84
Varicella zoster encephalitis 6
vasculitis 106
vasopressin *see* antidiuretic hormone
ventricular ectopic beats *81*, 82, *169*, 170
    in hypokalaemia *13*, 14
ventricular tachycardia *199*, 200
    atrial flutter with *43*, 44
villous adenoma 62
viral hepatitis 113, 114
visual loss 189, 190
    transient 141
vitamin B_{12} deficiency 46
vitamin D
    deficiency 172
    resistant (hypophosphataemic) rickets 137, 138
vitamin K deficiency 172

warfarin 192
Waterhouse–Friedrichsen syndrome 158
Wegener's granulomatosis 146
Wilson's disease 174
Wolff-Chaikoff effect 36
Wolff–Parkinson–White syndrome *47*, 48

zidovudine 181, 182
Zieve's syndrome 10